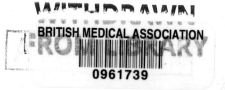

Part 3 MRCOG

Your Essential Revision Guide

Part 3 MRCOG

Your Essential Revision Guide

LISA JOELS

Consultant Obstetrician and Gynaecologist,
Royal Devon and Exeter NHS Foundation Trust

EDMUND NEALE

Consultant Obstetrician and Gynaecologist,
Bedford Hospital NHS Trust and Milton Keynes University Hospital

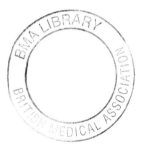

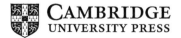
CAMBRIDGE
UNIVERSITY PRESS

CAMBRIDGE
UNIVERSITY PRESS

University Printing House, Cambridge CB2 8BS, United Kingdom

Cambridge University Press is part of the University of Cambridge.

It furthers the University's mission by disseminating knowledge in the pursuit of
education, learning and research at the highest international levels of excellence.

www.cambridge.org
Information on this title: www.cambridge.org/9781316627457

© Cambridge University Press 2016

First published 2016

Printed in the United Kingdom by Clays, St Ives plc

A catalogue record for this publication is available from the British Library

ISBN 978-1-316-62745-7 Paperback

Contents

Foreword

Membership of the Royal College of Obstetricians and Gynaecologists (RCOG) is recognised worldwide as certifying a high standard of clinical skills, and carries significant prestige. The MRCOG examination is an exacting test of those clinical skills comprising three parts. In each part of the exam applied clinical knowledge is assessed and a sound understanding of the evidence base underpinning the practice of obstetrics and gynaecology is essential. Clinical practice involves face-to-face contact with patients, and therefore the ability to demonstrate knowledge and skills in real-life encounters is fundamental to working as an obstetrician and gynaecologist.

Practising obstetrics and gynaecology to a high standard is not just about knowledge, however. Our mothers and patients can be well informed and often wish to be involved in making decisions about the care they and their babies receive, so the good obstetrician and gynaecologist will also have good communication skills, while keeping the safety of patients at the forefront of their minds.

As experienced teachers and examiners, we have seen able doctors fail the clinical assessment, not because of a lack of knowledge, but due to poor exam technique, failure to understand the skills being tested and by making simple errors. We hope that this book and its linked video resources will give you the chance to practise the skills needed to demonstrate in the exam setting the skills that you routinely use every day. We also hope that the detailed discussions of the marking schemes will show you how to pass each task in the Part 3 exam.

We couldn't have prepared this revision resource without the help of a large team. We'd like to thank Chris Chivers, Head of Examinations, who has provided editorial input and detailed advice about the style and structure of the book. Karen Penfold has contributed to the typing of large sections of the book in addition to helping with many other RCOG activities over a long period of time.

We'd like to thank the team who helped create the video resources. Christine Tang, Part 3 MRCOG Administrator, and Helen Munn, eLearning Manager, organised and managed the filming of the video resources with precision and patience. Colin Duncan, Paul Mills and Lesley Briggs brought their experience of being involved as examiners to the simulated tasks and in providing detailed examiner's comments for the book, which give an important insight as to how examiners make their judgements. We are very grateful to the team of junior doctors who were prepared to simulate both good and poor performance in the scenarios: Alex Tan, Vishalli Ghai, Kim Nash, Catherine Langley, Kathryn Tompsett, Sadia Hussain, James McLaren and Maryam Modarres.

Finally, we'd like to thank Andrew Starks at the RCOG for his patience and skills in recording and editing the videos.

We do hope that you find this resource valuable and that it helps you to show the examiners all your skills on the day of the exam in order to pass the membership examination. Good luck.

Lisa Joels and Edmund Neale

1 The Part 3 Clinical Assessment in the Context of the MRCOG Examination

This revision guide addresses the knowledge, skills, attitudes and competencies needed in preparation for the Part 3 MRCOG clinical assessment (the Part 3 exam). By using this book and the accompanying video resources at an early stage, exam candidates will have the best chance of honing their core clinical skills in preparation for the Part 3 exam. This chapter starts with a very brief summary of all three elements of the MRCOG examination. Further details can be found on the RCOG website (www.rcog. org.uk/en/careers-training/mrcog-exams).

The Format of the MRCOG Examination

The MRCOG examination consists of three parts and is set at the standard of a competent year-five specialty trainee (ST5). In training in obstetrics and gynaecology in the UK, the transition from ST5 to ST6 marks the completion of core training and the start of advanced skills training prior to the certificate of completion of training (CCT) at the end of ST7, and the move to independent practice as a consultant. A UK trainee who has completed five years of structured training should be able to manage the majority of problems encountered on the delivery suite, most common gynaecological emergencies and be able to run general gynaecological and antenatal clinics with minimal or indirect supervision. In addition, an ST5 trainee will have a working knowledge of most subspecialist practice even if they cannot manage those cases independently. Figure 1.1 shows the position of the Part 3 MRCOG examination within the UK Specialty Training Programme.

Over the years, the format of the examination has changed a number of times in line with developments in postgraduate medical education in order to ensure that the examination remains a rigorous assessment of competence. Each change is approved by the General Medical Council (GMC) and based in sound educational theory. The MRCOG examination is rigorously quality assured on an ongoing basis by the Examination and Assessment Committee and the Education Quality Assurance Committee.

The current format of the MRCOG examination consists of three parts, each of which was extensively piloted and analysed before being approved by the GMC and implemented.

The Part 1 MRCOG examination may be attempted at any stage of training after obtaining a medical degree. The Part 1 exam consists of two papers each lasting

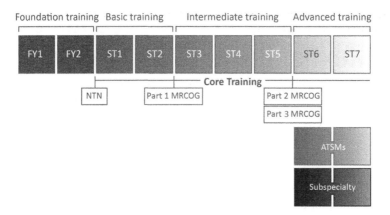

Figure 1.1 The position of the Part 3 MRCOG examination within the UK Specialty Training Programme.

2.5 hours and containing 100 single best answer (SBA) questions. The questions assess applied clinical sciences as defined in the Part 1 curriculum, which is available on the RCOG website. In UK training, Part 1 must be passed in order for the trainee to move from basic to intermediate training (ST2 to ST3).

The Part 2 MRCOG examination may be attempted once a trainee has passed the Part 1 exam and met the training requirements as specified on the RCOG website. Those doctors wishing to become a UK consultant must attempt Part 2 for the first time within seven years of passing the Part 1 examination (or ten years pro rata for less than full-time trainees or doctors not wishing to join the GMC specialist register). The format of the examination is two papers, each of which is three hours long and consists of 50 SBAs and 50 extended matching questions (EMQs).

The Part 3 exam may only be attempted after passing the Part 2 exam. The Part 3 exam is a clinical assessment of knowledge, skills, attitudes and competencies. Passing the Part 3 examination leads to the award of the Membership of the Royal College of Obstetricians and Gynaecologists (MRCOG) and remains the essential waypoint for UK trainees to pass from core training to higher training (ST6 and ST7).

The Knowledge and Skills Being Assessed in the Part 3 MRCOG Examination

The Part 3 exam consists of 14 tasks which are linked to 14 of the knowledge-based modules in the UK obstetrics and gynaecology curriculum. The 14 modules of the Part 3 exam and the link to the respective module of the core curriculum are shown in Table 1.1.

A detailed description of the knowledge criteria for each of these modules is to be found in the core curriculum on the RCOG website.[1] Chapter 3 of this book

---

[1] www.rcog.org.uk/en/careers-training/specialty-training-curriculum/core-curriculum/

Table 1.1 The 14 modules of the Part 3 exam and the link to the respective module of the core curriculum

	Part 3 module name	Corresponding core curriculum module
1	Teaching	2 (teaching part only)
2	Core surgical skills	5
3	Post-operative care	6
4	Antenatal care	8
5	Maternal medicine	9
6	Management of labour	10
7	Management of delivery	11
8	Postpartum problems (the puerperium)	12
9	Gynaecological problems	13
10	Subfertility	14
11	Sexual and reproductive health	15
12	Early pregnancy care	16
13	Gynaecological oncology	17
14	Urogynaecology and pelvic floor problems	18

describes how the knowledge criteria for each module will be tested in the Part 3 exam.

Each of the Part 3 modules is assessed in the context of five domains:

1 patient safety
2 communication with patients and their relatives
3 communication with colleagues
4 information gathering
5 applied clinical knowledge

Each task will assess three or four of the domains to reflect everyday clinical practice where, for example, communicating with patients is inextricably linked with applied clinical knowledge, or communicating with colleagues also involves aspects of patient safety.

Chapter 2 of this book describes the professional behaviours being assessed in each of the five domains.

Practical Arrangements

The examination consists of a circuit of 14 tasks, each relating to one of the 14 modules to be assessed. Each task will be 12 minutes in length, which includes two minutes of initial reading time.

There may be several circuits running simultaneously in the London centre on each day of the examination and there may also be overseas centres.

The tasks in the morning and afternoon sessions will be the same, but there will be different tasks for each day of the examination. Candidates from the morning circuits will be kept separate from the afternoon candidates to ensure that the second cohort don't have an unfair advantage.

At the start of each task, candidates will have two minutes outside the booth to read the background information and instructions for the task. The buzzer will then sound and candidates will enter the booth and have ten minutes to complete the task. The information displayed outside the booth will be duplicated inside the booth, usually affixed to the desk.

> **Tip:** This isn't a test of short-term memory, so if you've forgotten the name or age of the patient etc., you can glance down at the information to remind you. More importantly, you should not be spending your valuable two minutes of reading time copying down information outside the booth when you should be preparing to show the examiner your skills.

There are two types of task in the Part 3 MRCOG: **simulated patient or colleague** tasks where the candidate interacts with an actor and **structured discussion** tasks in which the candidate interacts with the examiner. Marking is carried out in real time to ensure that no marks are forgotten and there is no recall bias. At the end of ten minutes, the buzzer sounds again and candidates move to the next task, where they again have two minutes to read the background information and instructions, and so on until all 14 tasks have been completed. The duration of the examination is slightly under three hours.

The purpose of the Part 3 MRCOG exam is to assess the skills that are expected of an ST5 in the clinical practice of obstetrics and gynaecology. The examination there-fore tests, in a fair and reproducible way, how candidates behave with patients and col-leagues, as well as how obstetrics and gynaecology is practised in the NHS.

> **Tip:** You may find it helpful to view the simulated patient tasks as being similar to seeing patients on the wards and in clinics, and the structured discussion tasks as being similar to either case-based discussions with your consultant or clinical governance tasks.

Simulated Patient or Colleague Tasks

In simulated patient tasks, candidates interact with an actor who has been trained and fully briefed in the role they are to play. They will know all the relevant details pertaining to the case and will have some scripted questions to prompt you if needed. They will show emotions such as anger, anxiety or distress if it is appropriate to the scenario; however, they won't display extreme behaviours such as shouting or swearing and they won't leave the station during the ten minutes of your examination.

Tip: It is often not possible to match the physical characteristics of the actors to the demographic and characteristics of the role they are playing. You may, for example, encounter a young actor in her twenties playing a 45-year-old woman with a gynaecological problem or vice versa. Similarly, your task might say the patient weighs 140 kg, but this is not reflected in the physical characteristics of the actor. It is therefore vital to read the background details of the case carefully and conduct the task according to the written instructions, not the apparent characteristics of the actor. Remember, these instructions will be affixed to the desk inside the station.

In a simulated patient (or colleague) task the examiner(s) will be 'a fly on the wall', meaning that they are observing the task and awarding marks but will take no part in it. They will have a neutral facial expression and will be making notes throughout the task. Candidates must not attempt to interact with the examiner by explaining things to them or asking them questions. It might help to imagine that they are the healthcare assistant (HCA) sitting in the gynaecology clinic. The HCA's role is to be a chaperone and not to interfere with the consultation or to interrupt. Candidates are advised to regard the examiner in exactly the same way as an HCA and only interact with the role player.

Tip: Don't forget to introduce yourself to the actor and address her or him by name. Communication skills will be covered in more detail in the next chapter.

Structured Discussion Tasks

In structured discussion tasks, candidates interact directly with a clinical examiner who will have detailed instructions about the task and a list of questions that they can use to prompt the candidate or to move the task on to ensure the candidate does not run out of time. The examiner may give the candidate further information (e.g. results of investigations or more clinical details) as the scenario evolves and then ask further questions. They may also ask the candidate to explain or expand on an answer. It may help to think of a structured discussion task as being similar to a handover, presenting a patient on a ward round or phoning a consultant out of hours. These are conversations that happen every working day, where information is exchanged and the consultant clarifies details or asks for further information where necessary.

Tip: The examiner's role is to ensure that all candidates with the necessary knowledge, skills, attitudes and competencies pass the MRCOG examination. It is widely assumed that examiners are there to fail candidates, when in fact the opposite is true. All examiners are trained to ensure that candidates are given the opportunity to demonstrate their skills. Examiners appreciate how stressful such a high-stakes examination is and want to help candidates overcome their nerves to perform at their best and achieve the marks they deserve. Don't assume that you are doing badly if the examiner moves you on; they are trying to ensure that you are able to cover all aspects of the scenario in the time available so that you have the best chance to demonstrate all your skills.

Linked Tasks

In addition to each task corresponding to a module from the above list, tasks may also be linked in some way. For example, there could be a task about intrapartum management (module 7) with an evolving scenario resulting in an adverse event such as a caesarean hysterectomy, which then could be linked to postnatal care (module 8) in the next task where issues of clinical governance are addressed or the patient needs to be debriefed. It is important to understand that although the scenarios are linked, the tasks will be marked independently and the two examiners will not discuss a candidate's performance. A poor performance in the first task, for example, will not affect the marks awarded in the second task.

Examiners

All Part 3 examiners have been formally trained in how to assess the skills, award the marks and conduct the examination. Prior to each examination there is a detailed examiner briefing at which all the examiners marking a particular task meet to review the instructions, the scenario and the marking scheme. This detailed training session ensures that each candidate is assessed against the same criteria and level of skills, irrespective of which circuit or examination centre they are allocated to. Similarly, there is also a detailed briefing and rehearsal for the simulated patients to ensure that they fully understand the role they are to play as defined in their instructions and to ensure that they perform their tasks in the same way and to the same standard in each circuit or examination centre.

Clinical Examiners

All clinical examiners are Fellows or Members of the RCOG in current clinical practice, selected through an appointments process and required to undertake a training programme. They understand the level of knowledge, skills and competencies of an ST5 trainee and are skilled in assessing whether candidates have the appropriate professional attitudes and behaviours to pass the MRCOG examination.

The examination is marked in real time. Notable aspects of the candidate's performance are documented as the task progresses and in the two minutes at the end of each task. The standard required to achieve a pass in each of the tasks and domains assessed is agreed before the start of the examination at an examiner briefing. Each examiner is provided with individual feedback on their performance in the examination as part of the quality assurance of the examination.

Lay Examiners

The involvement of lay examiners in the assessment of doctors is reflective of the contemporary approach to obstetrics and gynaecology in which patients are expected to be partners in their own care and to be involved in shared decision-making about their condition and any management plans. Lay examiners are recruited from the general public and do not have any clinical training or background, in order to ensure that they accurately represent the vast majority of patients that obstetricians and gynaecologists encounter on a daily basis. In at least four of the simulated patient tasks in any single exam there will be both a clinical and a lay examiner present.

The task of lay examiners is to mark the communication skills of the candidates in their interaction with patients and/or their families, as represented by the actors. They attend the briefing and rehearsal sessions for the task they will be examining, along with the clinical examiners and actors. As with clinical examiners, they award marks in real time during the task and in the two minutes after the candidate has left the booth. They do not discuss their marks with the clinical examiner, nor do they modify those marks after the candidate has left the booth.

All lay examiners have undergone an initial recruitment and selection process as well as a rigorous training programme to understand their role within the Part 3 MRCOG examination. All examiners are required to undertake equality and diversity training.

The Examination Blueprint

Each of the MRCOG examinations (Part 1, Part 2 and Part 3) are blueprinted separately to ensure that each module of the core curriculum is assessed at an appropriate level in each exam. Examples of the blueprints for each part of the examination are on the RCOG website.[2]

In the Part 3 examination, all 14 modules will be represented in every exam. Unlike the previous arrangement where the Part 2 written and oral exams shared a common blueprint, the Part 3 clinical assessment stands separately. The purpose of this is to ensure that the MRCOG examination as a whole is a thorough and comprehensive test of clinical knowledge and its application.

In the past, the Part 2 Oral Assessment contained similar topics on each day to fulfil the shared blueprinting requirements. The Part 3 exam is different. Each day of the Part 3 exam will be set and marked completely independently, with no links between the questions other than the modules from which they come. Thus, candidates on each day of the examination will have no prior knowledge of how each module may be tested. Each of the 14 modules will be tested with a separate task, so it is essential to have revised all the required subject areas.

Standard Setting

The Part 2 and Part 3 MRCOG examinations are criterion referenced against the level of an ST5 trainee, meaning that the standard required to pass remains consistent between examinations regardless of the relative difficulty of a particular examination.

---

[2] www.rcog.org.uk/globalassets/documents/careers-and-training/mrcog-exam/part-2/p2-blueprinting-grid.pdf

The level of knowledge and skills required in the Part 3 exam is that of a specialty trainee at level 5 (ST5), who has completed core and intermediate training. Each task will assess a minimum of three core clinical skill domains. For each domain being assessed, the examiner will be required to assess a candidate's performance as either Pass, Borderline or Fail. The judgements will be converted into numerical scores, which will then be used to calculate the candidate's mark. It is important to understand that this is a compensatory approach meaning that no single domain has greater importance than any other.

Medical training has been likened to a spiral in which subjects are first covered in breadth at medical school and then with an increasingly narrow focus as doctors specialise and increase their depth of knowledge to the level of a generalist at first, then a specialist and finally an expert. The syllabus for the MRCOG defines the knowledge level expected for each part of the curriculum and clearly shows that some areas will require significantly more in-depth knowledge than others.[3] For example, management of pre-eclampsia is a routine part of practice in obstetrics, which trainees will encounter repeatedly during a working week and therefore will be expected to have a high level of knowledge and skills in this area. In contrast, disorders of puberty are relatively uncommon and so trainees would be expected to have a sound theoretical knowledge but have less hands-on experience of managing such cases.

The MRCOG examination assesses knowledge and skills relating to both common and less common conditions and therefore some topics will be inherently more complex than others. This is dealt with in an examination by standard setting. The standard expected for each question or task will be set according to how difficult it is. The standard for a task relating to the management of pre-eclampsia, for example, will be higher than that for a task relating to precocious puberty as defined by the skill level of an ST5 specified in the syllabus. Standard setting ensures that if a trainee sat every diet of the examination, they would have the same chance of passing because for each examination the passing standard will be based on a combination of their skills and how difficult the exam is. The clinical examiners are all in current practice as consultants in obstetrics and gynaecology and therefore have a good understanding of what a competent ST5 should know and be able to do. This means that the passing standard may be different on each day of the examination, but candidates will stand the same chance of passing irrespective of which day they appear.

Quality Assurance

The RCOG makes every effort to ensure that all parts of the membership examination are developed and delivered fairly, in line with the latest evidence-based research. In the Part 3 exam, particular attention is given to consistency between circuits and between the two diets of the examination in May and November each year. There is a careful checking process to ensure that all examination material is accurate. The training and

---

[3] www.rcog.org.uk/en/careers-training/mrcog-exams/part-2-mrcog/syllabus

performance of examiners is assessed to ensure that examiners' marking is consistent and standardised. There is also a transparent appeals process for candidates who feel that they were not given the opportunity to demonstrate their skills.

Why Do Candidates Fail the Part 3 Exam?

It is inevitable that some candidates will be disappointed to find that they have not passed the clinical examination. This is rarely due to a lack of knowledge as these candidates would have already passed two written examinations. In this situation it is usually one of two problems: either the candidate has allowed the stress of the examination to affect their performance, or they have been unable to demonstrate the required core clinical skills. In the first case, these candidates need to practise and rehearse, especially in relation to time management. They should consider accessing face-to-face courses to build their confidence. In the second case, working through the chapters of this book, including the written and video examples, should provide useful guidance in improving their skills in order to succeed.

Additional Resources

Anastasi A (1976) *Psychological Testing*, 4th edition. Macmillan Publishing, New York.
Blueprint: www.rcog.org.uk/globalassets/documents/careers-and-training/mrcog-exam/part-2/p2-blueprinting-grid.pdf
Curriculum: www.rcog.org.uk/en/careers-training/specialty-training-curriculum/core-curriculum/
General Medical Council: www.gmc-uk.org
MRCOG exams: www.rcog.org.uk/en/careers-training/mrcog-exams
Royal College of Obstetricians and Gynaecologists: www.rcog.org.uk
Syllabus: www.rcog.org.uk/en/careers-training/mrcog-exams/part-2-mrcog/syllabus

2 Core Clinical Skills

In order to practise safe obstetrics and gynaecology as a senior trainee and ultimately as an independent practitioner, it is essential to have a thorough and comprehensive understanding of obstetrics and gynaecology, including the evidence base underpinning this knowledge. The MRCOG examination has consistently been shown to be an excellent assessment of the knowledge required to move from core to higher training. The knowledge that will be assessed by the MRCOG examination is clearly defined in the MRCOG curriculum and has not changed despite alterations in the structure of the exam.

There is much more to the practice of clinical medicine than being really clever and having a comprehensive knowledge of anatomy, physiology and pathology. The practice of clinical medicine requires an understanding of how to apply clinical knowledge to an individual patient and, in modern medicine, also requires a patient-centred approach. The General Medical Council (GMC) has identified that deficiencies in pure knowledge are seldom the reason for patients' complaints or referral to the GMC's fitness-to-practice panel. Therefore this demonstrates that becoming a senior medical practitioner is about more than pure acquisition of knowledge. It includes being able to apply those core clinical skills, competencies and attitudes to each individual patient in a framework based on safety and team working. These additional skills are defined in the curriculum and are assessed by a combination of workplace-based assessments and the MRCOG examination. The Part 1 and Part 2 MRCOG exams have been shown to be robust assessments of core and applied clinical knowledge.

The Part 3 MRCOG exam tests those same core clinical skills in the context of a patient-centred knowledge and skills framework to ensure that passing candidates have the necessary skills to move to higher training and independent practice. Throughout the Part 3 exam, the clinical and lay examiners are asked to identify the 'competent candidate' and they are given detailed descriptions about the skills that a competent candidate would be expected to demonstrate. The importance of understanding this is that they aren't looking for a 'good' or 'excellent' candidate and the passing standard isn't set at an unreasonable level.

This chapter will define the five core clinical skills as introduced in the previous chapter and explain how they will be assessed in the Part 3 exam. As you will see, while these five core clinical skills or domains are explicit within the Part 3 assessment template, within any individual clinical scenario or task they will be intimately entwined.

Patient Safety

This clinical skill is arguably the most important in the modern-day practice of obstetrics and gynaecology. The practice of obstetrics in the UK has an enviable history of continuous improvement based on the longest running clinical audit of practice in the form of the triennial confidential enquiries. This has resulted in incremental reductions in maternal mortality rates right up to the present day. A similar approach to fetal and neonatal safety is now being driven through the MBBRACE database. With increasing specialisation in gynaecology there is good evidence that better outcomes are achieved when specific procedures are performed by specialists who have been appropriately trained and who continuously audit and benchmark their work. The emphasis on patient safety is reflected in the Part 3 exam and will be assessed in each of the 14 tasks, albeit by different methods. The GMC makes clear the importance of both patient safety and dignity throughout their document *Good Medical Practice*. So, given that patient safety is so pivotal to the way obstetrics and gynaecology is practised in the UK, why do some candidates, who clearly have the required knowledge, fail the clinical assessment in the domain of patient safety?

Common pitfalls:

- Not understanding the role of clinical governance in promoting patient safety.
- Not understanding the use of audit in identifying trends and systematic problems.
- Not understanding the duty of candour to provide apologies and explanations when care falls short of expected standards.

The GMC document *Good Medical Practice* is a really useful starting point for understanding the fundamental importance of patient safety. The GMC explicitly states that doctors should recognise the limits of their clinical ability and refer or call for help appropriately. Candidates attempting the Part 3 exam should have a clear understanding of the role of the ST5 trainee and the circumstances in which they would be expected to call for help. A candidate who, in the examination, fails to take any responsibility for decision-making and persistently defers to 'their consultant' is as likely to fail the patient safety domain as those candidates who do not mention involving senior staff at an appropriate time. The reality is that often as an ST5 you will have called for help but the senior team will be coming into the hospital so you would be expected to demonstrate your ability to cope while help is on the way. A good analogy for this is a cardiac arrest situation in which the practitioner has called for help but would be expected to start basic life support while the 'arrest team' is making its way to the bedside. When you take the Part 3 exam you need to be able to demonstrate to the examiner that you understand the limitations of your experience, call for help at an appropriate time, and are able to cope under pressure while waiting for help to arrive.

Confidentiality is paramount in caring for patients and patient information is protected by the *Data Protection Act* (DPA). Healthcare professionals have a duty to ensure that identifying information about patients is kept confidential and each healthcare organisation has a Caldicott Guardian to ensure appropriate safeguards are in place. All parts of the patient record, including paper notes, electronic notes and images, are covered by the DPA. Your understanding about confidentiality may be assessed in the Part 3 exam in a number of ways. A task may require a root cause analysis of an incident which resulted in a breach of confidentiality. The competent candidate will understand the implications of a breach of confidentiality both for the patient and the organisation. They will have an understanding of the clinical governance processes involved. You should therefore have a clear understanding of the principle of duty of candour and the need to explain and apologise for a breach of confidentiality in a simulated patient scenario but you should also appreciate the need to avoid criticising or undermining the colleague involved.

The competent candidate will understand that family members, including a spouse, do not have the right to know confidential information about a patient unless she has given consent. This includes issues relating to contraception, care in pregnancy and termination of pregnancy. It is essential that you understand the principles of mental capacity as defined in both the *Mental Capacity Act* and in terms of Lord Fraser competency for girls aged 13–18 years seeking contraceptive advice or termination of pregnancy. A good understanding of how to obtain informed consent is an essential skill and is likely to be tested in the Part 3 exam.

Patient safety includes a respect for patient dignity at all times and candidates should ensure that chaperones are used for intimate examinations. In the Part 3 exam it would be essential to explain the need for a chaperone. If, for example, you were teaching a trainee how to do a vaginal examination or gynaecological procedure you should tell them about the need for a chaperone so the examiner can note it on the mark sheet.

Another feature of patient dignity is a respect for the patient's religious beliefs and cultural issues. The competent candidate will understand that a Jehovah's Witness will not accept red cell transfusions and other blood fractions from donated blood even if refusal will result in their death. If the task involves a Jehovah's Witness, you should establish precisely what blood products the patient will accept, including cell salvage blood, and agree a management plan that respects the patient's beliefs.

A respect for cultural issues, however, does not allow patients to break UK law and the competent candidate will understand the need to report cases of female genital mutilation (FGM) and consider the safeguarding issues of the children or siblings of women affected by FGM. Since October 2015, it has been mandatory for healthcare professionals to inform the police of cases of FGM. You should also ensure that you understand how to deal with disclosures of domestic abuse and safeguarding issues. Every healthcare organisation in the UK will have a named nurse and doctor for safeguarding of children and vulnerable adults. Tasks featuring safeguarding issues in both adults and children are likely to feature in the Part 3 exam.

Despite clinical governance being a cornerstone of the practice of obstetrics and gynaecology in the UK for many years, adverse events continue to happen. Risk management includes developing protocols and policies to minimise adverse events and in particular 'never events' such as wrong-site surgery, transfusion of blood of the wrong blood group and prescribing errors including allergies, teratogenicity and interactions. The World Health Organization has developed a safe surgery checklist which is now in use throughout the NHS and candidates must be familiar with how this is used in theatres to reduce the risk of adverse events, particularly in emergency situations such as category one caesarean sections and ruptured ectopic pregnancy. The Part 3 exam could include a structured discussion about safe surgery.

Prescribing errors are thought to occur in up to 10 per cent of hospital admissions across all specialties. In obstetrics there are particular issues about safe prescribing in terms of teratogenicity, trans-placental transfer of drugs, excretion via breast milk and awareness of altered doses and regimens according to body mass index. In gynaecology there are specific issues about drug interactions which might reduce the efficacy of contraceptive methods; throughout both specialties, candidates need to be aware of the prescribing issues for patients with allergies or renal impairment. The task could include prescribing, so you should be able to safely and accurately complete a prescription chart for drugs and intravenous fluids, taking into account the individual patient's clinical condition. You should be familiar with the doses, routes of administration and risks or side-effects of the commonly used drugs in obstetrics and gynaecology. This will include prescribing antibiotics to patients with penicillin allergy due to the emphasis on sepsis in the most recent Confidential Enquiry into Maternal Death (MBBRACE).

Both treatments and investigations pose threats to patients in the form of complications even when the procedure has been carried out entirely correctly. In order to ensure patient safety, the correct checks must be done before an intervention, and you must understand the importance of excluding pregnancy before undertaking procedures involving ionising radiation or procedures on the uterus such as hysteroscopy or hysterectomy.

The practice of obstetrics and gynaecology places competing demands on a doctor's time, and the ability to triage the urgency of those demands is an essential skill both for working under pressure and for ensuring patient safety so that the patients with the greatest need wait the shortest time for attention. There are a number of ways that the skill of triage and prioritisation could be assessed in terms of patient safety in the Part 3 exam. A task could include a need to prioritise patients with gynaecological problems to identify those needing to be on the urgent suspected cancer (two-week wait) pathway. You could be asked to prioritise workload for an on-call shift either on labour ward or with gynaecological emergencies. The GMC makes it clear that at all times doctors should be prepared to explain and justify their decision-making and actions, even if their recommendations are not completely in line with established evidence due to the patient's wishes or other illnesses. You should be able to demonstrate your ability to work under pressure and be able to make and justify decisions based on the principles of triage and patient safety.

The GMC stipulates that doctors must take steps to monitor and improve the quality of their work, so you should have a good understanding of how audit, reflective practice, workplace-based assessments and the use of a logbook or portfolio can fulfil these requirements.

Suggestions for Developing Patient Safety Skills

- Spend some time reviewing RCOG guidelines on obtaining consent.
- Thoroughly revise the guidelines about assessing mental capacity and Lord Fraser competency.
- Practise writing prescriptions, drug charts and intravenous fluid administration charts, and ask your exam buddy to check they are correct and legible.
- Learn the doses and administration protocols for drugs commonly used in obstetrics and gynaecology.
- Make sure you are familiar with national guidance such as the WHO safe surgery checklist.
- Review both adult and child safeguarding principles and processes.
- Think about how audit, protocols and adverse-event reporting influences your every-day practice.

Communication with Patients and Families

Communication with patients and, from time to time, their families is a fundamental skill for all doctors in clinical practice. Doctors need to be able to explain the conditions from which patients are suffering, discuss investigations and treatment options and ultimately obtain informed consent from their patients. The ability to build relationships with patients in a very short space of time when patients are often at their most stressed and most vulnerable is a skill particularly needed in obstetrics and gynaecology. Doctors may meet the patient and their family for the first time in a crisis such as a stillbirth, fetal distress requiring a category one caesarean section or following a collapse from a ruptured ectopic pregnancy.

In many of the encounters doctors have with patients in obstetrics and gynaecology, patients are generally well and do not want to conform to the 'sick patient' role. This is particularly the case with obstetric patients and patients making contraceptive choices. Communication with patients therefore requires a different level of skills, including the ability to inform, engage, negotiate and make shared decisions. Given that communication with patients forms the biggest part of a doctor's working day, why do candidates with the clinical knowledge to pass the written element of the MRCOG examination then fail the Part 3 exam?

Common pitfalls:

- Candidates forget to introduce themselves and explain their role.
- Making assumptions about risk-taking behaviour.
- Feeling awkward or embarrassed about asking questions about lifestyle.
- Telling patients what they need rather than negotiating a plan.
- Not listening to the patient or respecting their views.
- Using unnecessary jargon, abbreviations or euphemisms that the patient does not understand.

The start of any clinical encounter is an introduction so that the patient and/or their family knows who they are speaking to and what that person's role is. In 2015 in the UK there was a national campaign to encourage all healthcare professionals to open a conversation with patients by saying 'Hello, my name is . . . '. It is therefore essential to do this in the Part 3 exam. It is up to the individual candidate to decide how they introduce themselves; are they going to say hello, I'm Dr Smith, Dr Jane Smith or Jane? The most sensible approach would be to introduce yourself in the examination exactly as you would in everyday clinical practice. You should then explain your role, for example: 'I'm the registrar/trainee in the clinic/labour ward today.' It may be that you have a different job title in everyday clinical practice, but for the purposes of the Part 3 exam you should call yourself the registrar (or ST5 trainee) since that is the level at which the examination is aimed. It's then vital to check the patient's name and establish what they would like you to call them, whether they are happy to be called by their first name or whether they would prefer to be called 'Mrs Jones', for example. As you read this paragraph, you are probably thinking that this advice is too basic, but you would be amazed how many candidates make this fundamental mistake due to a combination of nerves and a desire to get straight to the point of the task. Remember, the examiner, and in particular the lay examiner, will be making notes about your ability to engage with and develop a rapport with the simulated patient, and it's really hard to do this well if the actor doesn't know your name.

Communication is a two-way process and involves listening to the patient as well as giving them information. A good starting point is 'breaking the **ICE**' by listening to the patient's *Ideas, Concerns and Expectations*. It is essential in the Part 3 exam to give the simulated patient a chance at the start of the task to explain their ideas, concerns and expectations as they will have been given explicit instructions about what to say and do and this will guide you as to how to tackle the task going forwards.

Communication skills include verbal and non-verbal skills, so the examiners will be looking specifically for active listening, empathy and appropriate emotional responses. Active listening includes making and keeping eye contact, having an open posture and nodding or making encouraging sounds to indicate you are happy for the patient to keep talking. An open posture means avoiding crossing your arms in front of your body and ensuring you face the patient. In the Part 3 exam there will be a desk or table between you and the actor, which isn't best practice in the clinical setting; however, don't try to move the desk or your chair as the booths are often very small and you don't want to waste time or, even worse, knock over the partitions. Communication skills also include identifying barriers to communication, such as language barriers or disabilities. It's highly unlikely that use of interpreters would be assessed in the Part 3 exam.

Displaying empathy and appropriate emotional responses means taking a good look at your unconscious behaviours. Some people have a nervous laugh when they are stressed or under pressure, which is understandable but could be catastrophic if you are delivering bad news and then appearing to laugh at the situation. Some candidates seem to believe that they should always smile at the actor at the start of the task. While this shows that the candidate is friendly, this can be misconstrued as being unsympathetic if the task is breaking bad news, for which a solemn expression is more appropriate. Some excellent communicators can use humour or jokes to build rapport, but in the exam setting this is very risky and not advised. This advice may again seem to be very basic, but is based on observations of real candidates under exam conditions. Try videoing yourself or getting feedback from colleagues or your exam buddy to spot your unconscious behaviours.

The tasks assessing communication skills will be looking for an empathic, patient-centred approach. It is really important to look at the simulated patient's non-verbal cues as well as actively listening to them. A simulated patient who becomes evasive, looking away or shifting in their seat, is trying to give you a cue to ask more searching questions. This could be a cue to a situation of domestic violence, sexual abuse or coercion. A candidate showing empathy will pause briefly if the role player becomes tearful and will offer a tissue, or for a relative to join the discussion. Bear in mind that in the exam there won't be anyone to join and the role player won't waste time by spending the whole ten minutes sobbing – they are just trying to give you the opportunity to demonstrate your empathy.

Taking a relevant history forms part of the assessment of communication skills for many tasks in the Part 3 exam. This is discussed in more detail in the section on information gathering, but a common pitfall is for candidates to be obviously ill at ease when asking certain questions. There is no need to apologise for asking if a woman smokes or drinks alcohol; these are not illegal activities and no one will be offended by a simple enquiry. However, it is essential to avoid making assumptions about lifestyle choices of the patients portrayed in the tasks. The Part 3 exam will address sensitive areas such as sexually transmitted infections, contraceptive choices and termination of pregnancy, but you shouldn't assume that every simulated patient will be taking drugs or have multiple sexual partners. These assumptions will provoke distressed or angry reactions from the simulated patient and may derail your consultation. The examiners will be looking for a non-judgemental approach to the patient's concerns and decisions.

When giving information to a patient or their family, it is important to make sure that the patient isn't overwhelmed by information overload. Try to give information in 'chunks', small amounts of information after which you pause and check the patient has understood. Checking understanding can include a simple enquiry such as 'Is that okay?', or could be a brief pause to summarise what you have said and asking whether the patient has any questions. It's really important to encourage the patient to ask questions, because the role player will try to bring you back on track if you have strayed away from the focus of the task. They know what areas of discussion will award you marks on the examiner's mark sheet. This mimics real-life encounters in clinical situations in which healthcare professionals may be proud of their ability to make a management plan, but the patient leaves dissatisfied because they don't feel they have had their concerns addressed. Allow the simulated patient to guide you to their ideas, concerns and expectations as this is likely to allow you to gain marks and will improve your chance of gaining a pass in communication skills.

We now live in an information-rich society where the vast majority of people have access to the internet and patients are becoming increasingly well informed about healthcare issues. This has led to a rise in patients who want to be more involved in decision-making about their clinical problems and also about deciding, for example, their birth plans, where they may not fully appreciate the implications of their past medical, gynaecological or obstetric history. Such patients feel that they are experts in their own clinical condition and may have very firm or fixed ideas. Patients have the right to make decisions about themselves and the principle of autonomy ensures that if a patient has mental capacity, they have the right to make decisions about their care even if those decisions are unwise or against medical advice.

Communication tasks in the Part 3 exam will assess the ability of the candidate to avoid conflict and to negotiate with the patient to agree a safe plan. However, a safe plan is not always a textbook plan. Negotiating skills include demonstrating respect for the patient's views while providing information to either correct misunderstandings or to provide additional information that the patient may have been unaware of. Negotiating skills include being able to compromise where it is safe to do so, but not colluding with the patient to agree a plan that isn't safe. Doctors need to be able to explain the consequences of decisions against medical advice in a factual way to ensure patients have full information, but without antagonising the patient, which could result in a breakdown of communication and increase risks. It is essential that doctors are honest and don't overstate or exaggerate risks in order to force patients to comply with their plan of management. It is quite likely in the Part 3 exam that you will be asked to develop an agreed management plan for a patient that is safe, yet does not conform to standard practice or guidelines. Doctors must be honest in their communication with patients as issues of probity are a major concern for the GMC.

In clinical practice, doctors use medical terminology to ensure they are communicating accurately and clearly with colleagues; medical language is second nature to most medical practitioners. Patients, however, do not have a good understanding of most medical language, so the ability to translate medical jargon back to plain English is an essential communication skill. When talking to patients, choose your words carefully and use plain language wherever possible. Sometimes it is necessary to use medical terminology, but you should then explain what it means; for example, when taking consent for a total hysterectomy you can use the term but you should then explain verbally, and if necessary on the consent form, that this means removal of the 'womb and the neck of the womb'. This is especially important when explaining a diagnosis – for example, if a patient has endometriosis, it's important to tell them the term but you must then explain exactly what the condition is rather than assuming that all women will have heard of it.

Another common pitfall when trying to avoid using medical terminology is inappropriate use of euphemisms. It is acceptable to use terms like vagina and vulva rather than euphemisms such as 'down below', which could mean the vagina or could (technically) mean a lower floor in the building. Candidates often struggle to explain meconium staining of the liquor to the simulated patient. It's acceptable to explain that the baby has opened its bowels, but saying 'the baby has done a poo' is not advisable as this is the sort of language a parent would use to a child and would not normally use in adult conversation. In a task such as this, it is important to explain the implications of meconium staining and not assume that the patient knows why this is so concerning.

At the conclusion of any interaction with a patient or their family, it is essential to be able to summarise the discussion and then explain clearly a logical and reasoned plan for the next steps. This includes conveying short- and long-term plans, how results from tests will be communicated to the patient, discussing discharge from hospital, recovery and rehabilitation after surgery, and return to work. The encounter should always conclude with a final check that the patient has understood and by giving them a final opportunity to ask any questions.

Suggestions for Developing Communication Skills with Patients and Their Relatives

- Practise tasks with your exam buddy to improve non-verbal communication skills and unconscious behaviours.
- Practise 'chunking', breaking up information-giving into smaller, more manageable chunks.
- Rehearse asking difficult questions while maintaining a non-judgemental approach.
- Practise negotiating skills; for example, rehearse how you would counsel a patient wanting a homebirth after previous caesarean section.
- Think about medical terminology and decide which terms you will use with explanation, and which you will replace with non-medical language when talking to patients. It's then essential to practice this before the exam.

Communication with Colleagues

Communication skills are so important that they will be assessed in most of the 14 tasks by both clinical and lay examiners. This could be either communication with patients, their families or with clinical colleagues.

Modern obstetrics and gynaecology involves shift work and working within a multi-disciplinary team. This means that the ability to communicate with medical, nursing and midwifery colleagues safely at handover, via the notes for both inpatients and out-patients and with colleagues in primary care is an essential skill for senior trainees and doctors practising independently. This might involve the transfer of verbal or written information, taking into account UK law in terms of the Data Protection Act. Communication with colleagues needs to be succinct, relevant and to encompass the essential positive findings, relevant negative findings and outstanding tasks still to be completed in order to ensure that colleagues involved in subsequent care can develop an adequate care plan.

Communication is a fundamental part of teaching skills as well, and these will also be assessed in the Part 3 exam. Since no doctors work in complete isolation, and communication with colleagues in healthcare is part of everyday practice, it is surprising that candidates with the clinical knowledge to pass the written elements of the exam fall down on communication with colleagues in the Part 3 exam. In such a high-stakes examination, nerves often get the better of candidates and therefore it's really important that you develop excellent communication skills with colleagues so that your default behaviour under the pressure of exam conditions will meet the examiner's expectations.

Common pitfalls:

- Not adopting a logical, reasoned approach to clinical decision-making.
- Struggling to convey clear and succinct summaries.
- Failure to use a structured system of communication for handover such as the SBAR tool (*S*ituation, *B*ackground, *A*ssessment and *R*ecommendations) in order to ensure nothing is missed.
- Problems with writing legible, logical and ordered clinical notes, plans or operating notes.
- Not understanding the diverse roles and dynamics of a multidisciplinary team.

Tasks in the Part 3 exam will include an assessment of communication with colleagues in both verbal and written forms. Candidates will be expected to demonstrate their ability to convey information succinctly and in a logical and structured way. When you approach these tasks your summary of the history, examination and results of investigation should focus on the salient points and then be followed by a clear and well-reasoned plan. This is a different skill from information gathering as the ability to summarise and convey relevant information demonstrates the ability to think critically about what is important and why those facts need to be communicated. The Part 3 exam could include written tasks such as writing operation notes, preparing a letter to a GP, a referral to another specialty, a discharge summary or a prescription. The competent candidate will have clear, legible handwriting. There is a tendency for handwriting to become untidy when trying to write quickly, and with widespread use of computers and electronic systems to record notes, order investigations and prescribe drugs, it is easy to get out of the habit of writing. While in everyday clinical practice you may use a pen, in the Part 3 exam you will be given a pencil to use, so it would be helpful if you practise writing with one before you sit the exam. If you are making an entry in a patient's notes, always document the date, time, your name and role and then sign each entry. Always make a plan at the end of an entry in the notes, even if the plan is very simple, such as to review in 30 minutes or repeat the vaginal examination in four hours.

Writing prescriptions accurately and legibly tests both written communication and patient safety. It is really important to be able to do this task, and if you are unfamiliar with the style of charts used in the NHS, there is really useful information and examples of prescription charts on the website of the Academy of Medical Royal Colleges[1]. There is a strong focus in the NHS on appropriate antibiotic stewardship so any prescriptions for antibiotics should either have a stop date or a date when microbial sensitivities should be checked to confirm that the most appropriate drug is being used.

Writing clinic letters and referral letters to other specialties is a particular skill. The letter shouldn't duplicate information that was contained in the referral letter, but should

---

[1] http://www.aomrc.org.uk/publications/reports-guidance/standards-design-hospital-prescription-charts-0411/

contain any salient facts that have come to light during the consultation or examination and the results of any investigations along with a clear plan for treatment and/or follow-up. If the letter contains a task for the GP, such as prescribing medication or checking coil threads, this needs to be clear and stand out from the body of the letter. While the MRCOG is not a test of the English language, candidates should be familiar with the use of grammar, punctuation and paragraphs to ensure that the messages in the letter are clear.

Junior doctors in the NHS work in shifts of up to 12 hours; consultants may work shifts or be on call for 24 hours; and nurses and midwives usually work shifts of 8–12 hours. There are therefore a number of times during a 24-hour period when staff change and handover must occur to ensure that patient care continues seamlessly even though personnel have changed. Communication at handover is a core clinical skill, particularly on a labour ward and in relation to emergency admissions, and will be tested in the Part 3 exam. Safe and efficient handover includes a list of patients, where they are and a brief summary of their clinical situation. Handover will highlight high-risk patients who need review and whose clinical condition is at risk of deteriorating. The competent doctor will also hand over a list of tasks to be completed, such as blood results that are awaited and tasks they haven't been able to complete during their shift. While it is essential to give enough information at handover, there is also a skill in being succinct and keeping handover to relevant matters to ensure that the oncoming team isn't delayed in continuing with patient care. The handover process will also test the candidate's ability to triage and appropriately prioritise their workload. Handover may not be a familiar skill for doctors outside the area regulated by the European Working Time Directive and so they should familiarise themselves with the principles of handover as described by the GMC. Don't forget, within the Part 3 exam you may only have ten minutes to complete your handover, so you will need to think carefully about time management. If you spend eight minutes telling the examiner about the most straightforward of your patients you are unlikely to pass if you still have four more complex women to hand over.

It is essential to be able to communicate appropriately with all the healthcare professionals who make up the multidisciplinary team looking after women with obstetric or gynaecological problems. This team includes not only nurses working in traditional roles, but also nurses and midwives with clinical responsibilities of their own which dovetail with medical practitioners. Midwives are independent practitioners with responsibility for caring for women with uncomplicated pregnancy. The vast majority of pregnant women in the UK are cared for by midwives entirely throughout pregnancy and the postnatal period, without ever needing input from the medical team. Midwives are essential in identifying women developing complications of pregnancy who need to transition to consultant-led care and those women who are high-risk and need consultant-led care from the outset. Even those high-risk women under consultant-led care will still have considerable input from the midwives, and being able to communicate with, and provide care collaboratively with midwives is an essential skill which is founded on good communication skills. You should have a clear understanding of which tasks are appropriate to delegate to midwives or other members of the healthcare team, which tasks you should undertake yourself and when to call for senior help.

Other members of the team include specialist nurses, midwives and consultant midwives with extended roles providing direct care for patients working independently but alongside doctors. Their work is guided by protocols and standard operating procedures to ensure patient safety, and where clinical situations fall outside these protocols the nurse or midwife should refer the woman to the medical team. Examples of this are specialist midwives caring for women with safeguarding issues, drug and alcohol problems and complex mental health needs, specialist cancer nurses supporting the gynaecological oncology team, diabetes nurses supporting the medical antenatal team and specialist gynaecology nurses supporting the various formal Multidisciplinary Teams.

A common source of confusion is between the terminology referring to delivery of healthcare as multidisciplinary and the formal Multidisciplinary Team (MDT). Defining healthcare as multidisciplinary means including members of any of the disciplines from the administration team, nursing and allied health professionals, medical staff and the ancillary staff that run a hospital.

There are, however, a small number of formal MDTs. These include the gynaecological oncology team linking gynaecologists with pathologists, radiologists, radiotherapists, oncologists and specialist nurses. The medical antenatal MDT links obstetricians with physicians and specialist diabetes nurses. The urogynaecology teams in each Trust link with national databases in a virtual MDT. There are MDTs in endometriosis at a tertiary level linking gynaecologists with general, colorectal or urological surgeons, specialist nurses and administrators supporting national databases for these specialist teams of which there is usually only one per region in the UK. Understanding the complex nature of the structure of obstetric and gynaecological services makes it clear that communication with other clinical and non-medical staff is challenging as very few of these interactions will reflect the traditional and outdated view of the nurse as the doctor's handmaiden. Communication in these settings must reflect an understanding of, and respect for that person's role, training and expertise.

Communication-centred tasks in the Part 3 exam will assess team work and leadership skills. The tasks will include situations where you have to deal with clinical disagreement with medical, nursing or midwifery colleagues, including dealing sensitively with behavioural issues. The communication skills needed for this include actively listening to and respecting the views of colleagues, succinctly and with a logical approach explaining your view, being able to justify and explain your opinion and ultimately negotiating a plan of care which ensures patient safety.

Teaching junior colleagues is defined by the GMC as one of the core duties of a doctor. Teaching, either in the form of a tutorial, doing some bedside teaching such as a case-based discussion or in teaching a practical skill will be assessed in the Part 3 exam. The competent candidate will be able to demonstrate good communication by teaching with a logical coherent manner, recognising the skills of the learner and the resources available. You should understand the principles of adult learning and giving feedback.

Teaching a practical skill is a step-by-step process of demonstrating and explaining the task, asking the learner to explain the task back to the teacher and then finally getting the learner to demonstrate the skill. Communication should be clear and concise, consistent and show respect for the learner. Teaching includes giving feedback in a supportive, non-critical way by identifying good points before giving suggestions for improvement in specific areas. The competent candidate will invite the learner to ask questions and be willing to repeat instructions or give a reasoned justification in response to the learner's questions. A teaching session should conclude with an action plan for how the learner can improve and/or implement their new skills in practice. Throughout a teaching session there is a need to recognise patient safety and halt teaching or intervene if patient safety is at risk. The simulated trainee may be instructed to deliberately misunderstand or carry out a part of the procedure incorrectly to assess your ability to intervene without distressing or undermining the learner. Remember, however, in the Part 3 exam you will only have ten minutes, so you may have to describe some of the steps you would normally take briefly, to enable you to move through the task within the allotted time.

Suggestions for Developing Communication Skills with Colleagues

- Practise writing summaries and letters by hand and in pencil, especially if you use electronic notes at work.
- Reflect on clinic letters and discharge summaries written by your peers and senior colleagues to develop your own skills of letter writing.
- Ensure you understand the role of nurses and midwives in the UK.
- Practise scenarios where there is disagreement with colleagues over care plans.
- Get your exam buddy to watch you doing a timed teaching session.

Information Gathering

The skill of information gathering includes an understanding both of what information is needed and how to obtain that information. Taking a history is one of the first skills taught at medical school and remains the fundamental method of gathering information in order to construct a differential diagnosis and develop an appropriate management plan.

The competent candidate will be expected to elicit information from the actor depicting a simulated patient or trainee using a blend of mainly open and some closed questions. This is a skill that candidates are using every day in their work so it should be easy to achieve the required standard in each of the tasks, which begs the question why some candidates with the required level of knowledge to pass the Part 2 written papers fail the Part 3 exam on information gathering skills.

Common pitfalls:

- Wasting time by asking irrelevant questions.
- Asking mainly closed questions.
- Repeating questions/not listening to the answers.
- Ignoring cues from the actor.

Medical students are taught a template of the questions necessary to take a full obstetric or gynaecological history and they tend to follow this slavishly. Thus their histories are often cluttered with irrelevant facts – for example, asking a patient presenting with post-menopausal bleeding how old they were when they started their periods. Junior doctors starting their first post in obstetrics and gynaecology tend to follow a similar method of gathering information.

Using a standard or template approach to taking a history usually involves a long list of mainly closed questions. Closed questions are those that require a yes/no answer – for example, 'Do you have pelvic pain during sexual intercourse?' These questions close down discussion and make it very clear that the consultation is based on the doctor's agenda rather than the patient's expectations. A more appropriate approach is to use an open question – for example, 'Can you tell me what triggers your pelvic pain?' This allows the patient to guide the doctor to what matters most to her and what her underlying fears and concerns may be.

Practising obstetrics and gynaecology at a more senior level requires a different approach to history taking that demonstrates an understanding of clinical decision-making and the pathophysiology of disease. One way of taking a relevant and focused history is to use a Bayesian approach. Bayes theorem calculates pre-test probability and then uses a test to calculate the change in probability, the post-test probability, which determines whether the outcome is more or less likely. This is statistically presented as likelihood ratios, but this approach can also be used to take a structured history where the 'test' is a series of questions. Each question is used to determine whether a cause or pathology is more or less likely.

Experienced clinicians tend to start constructing a differential diagnosis very quickly after the start of the encounter with the patient. This could be from information in the referral letter from the general practitioner, or the response of the patient to an opening question such as 'How can I help you today?', or 'How are you? What seems to be the problem?' For example, if a teenage girl explains that she is experiencing pelvic pain, immediately a differential diagnosis will form in the clinician's mind. The clinician will then ask questions that make one diagnosis more or less likely, or rule a diagnosis in or out. Endometriosis is obviously one of the differential diagnoses in this scenario, so a careful enquiry about the timing of the pain in relation to the menstrual cycle demonstrates a targeted approach to history taking. The competent candidate will also draw on their knowledge that constipation and irritable bowel syndrome are also common conditions in teenagers, so their history will cover these non-gynaecological questions to rule these diagnoses in or out. If a sensitive enquiry about sexual partners reveals that the girl hasn't ever been sexually active, that effectively rules out sexually transmitted infections and means that requesting swabs from the vagina and cervix isn't a priority. Even more importantly, not asking a girl who has never been sexually active about dyspareunia shows the candidate has listened to the answers to the questions they asked and that they aren't doubting the truthfulness of those replies.

The actor in the Part 3 exam will not be briefed to mislead candidates by giving incorrect information or lying. They are given a very specific script and have been carefully briefed to ensure that they understand their symptoms and background so candidates can be confident in the truthfulness of the replies to their questions. The actor is instructed to give key clinical information to the candidate in response to open questions; the competent candidate should therefore ask open questions and use the answers to guide them as to what is likely to be on the examiner's mark sheet.

The GMC defines the duties of a doctor and states that doctors must be able to 'adequately assess the patient's conditions, taking account of their history (including the symptoms and psychological, spiritual, social and cultural factors), their views and values'. You should be able to gather information both about clinical problems and the wider issues relating to that patient in order to ensure a holistic, patient-centred approach to information gathering.

When preparing for the Part 3 exam, reflect on your own style of history taking. Are the majority of your questions open questions which allow the patient to explain their concerns and problems? Clinical practice in the real world is usually very busy, with competing demands on a doctor's time, and it's very tempting to default to closed questions to stop patients talking and move the consultation on more quickly. If you have slipped into this pattern at work, it's really important to prepare for the Part 3 exam by re-training yourself to ask mainly open questions. Work with a friend or exam buddy to practice information gathering and ask them to make a note of how many open or closed questions you ask. You can then review your approach to taking a history and practise ways to change this.

The competent candidate will use signposting to explain to the patient the structure of the consultation. For example: 'I appreciate that you are worried that you might have ovarian cancer but it would really help me if I could just ask you a few questions first before I explain the results of your scan.' This indicates to the patient (and the examiner) that you are aware of her concerns and you are going to address them with a patient-centred approach once you've obtained some key and focused information in which to frame your response to her concerns.

An integral part of information gathering is to use communication skills as discussed above. It's essential to adopt the correct body language and actively listen to the actor's answers to your questions. Only look down to make written notes if it's essential as this breaks eye contact with the simulated patient. Avoid repeating questions at all costs as it suggests you aren't listening to the answers. If you need to repeat the question because you haven't understood the actor, explain this to them by saying something like 'I'm sorry, I didn't understand that, could you explain what you meant please?' or something similar.

Information gathering isn't limited to just history taking and therefore candidates in a high-stakes postgraduate examination like the Part 3 exam can expect that other aspects of information gathering will also be assessed. A structured discussion task could include information gathering in the form of explaining which investigations are needed to investigate a clinical condition in order to make a diagnosis and develop a management plan. Previously in the Part 2 MRCOG oral assessment the structured mark sheet would have awarded marks as long as an investigation was mentioned, even without an explanation or justification. This encouraged candidates to adopt a scattergun approach of saying every investigation they could think of in order to gain marks. In the

Part 3 exam candidates are unlikely to achieve a pass if they adopt this approach. You should be able to explain what the relevant investigations are, ensuring that resources aren't wasted in over-investigation and that patients aren't exposed to unnecessary risks linked with invasive testing.

The tasks could include a writing task involving reviewing a clinical incident and making a plan of the approach to gather information in order to undertake a root cause analysis. Incident reporting is a key part of ensuring patient safety. A root cause analysis can identify systematic errors that can be corrected to minimise the risk of recurrence. It can also identify the need for additional training for specific individuals or the need to make available additional equipment, drugs or procedures. This is part of a no-blame culture which aims to avoid blaming individuals when systems fail, but also fosters a culture of individual responsibility for providing safe patient care. You should understand how to review documentation and be able to describe a plan for information gathering to contribute to the root cause analysis. Then you should be able to use the information collected in a root cause analysis to debrief or explain events to a patient or their family in an open and honest way without undermining colleagues.

The tasks may include information gathering in the form of interpreting the results of investigations, operations or cardiotocograph traces. You must be able to demonstrate a logical and clearly reasoned approach to these tasks in order to achieve a pass in the domain of information gathering.

Suggestions for Developing Information Gathering Skills

- Find someone to help you. You could work with a friend, relative, your partner or an exam buddy to help you with these practical skills. If all else fails, video yourself and critically appraise your own performance.
- Practise a few opening statements so they become second nature to you. For example: 'Hello, I'm Doctor X and I'm the registrar in clinic today. Can you tell me what has brought you here today?'
- Work with your exam buddy to practise open questions and reduce the number of closed questions you use so that your performance in the Part 3 exam is natural and unforced.
- Consider recording your practice attempts so you can reflect on your approach.
- Practise your signposting statements. For example: 'I've read your GP's letter and understand that you've been trying to get pregnant for two years. It would really help me if I could just ask a few questions before we discuss the next steps.'
- Get your exam buddy to listen to you taking a history and make a note of how many times you asked an irrelevant question or didn't pick up on the patient's cues.

It may be difficult or may feel embarrassing to practise in front of someone else, but if you choose an exam buddy that you trust, this rehearsal will be invaluable in reducing your exam stress and improving your performance (and that of your exam buddy) in the Part 3 exam.

Applied Clinical Knowledge

Clinical knowledge in the form of anatomy, physiology, biochemistry, pathology and pharmacology is the bedrock of studying medicine at both undergraduate and postgraduate level, but pure knowledge has limited value in the real world. The real importance of clinical knowledge is in understanding how to apply this knowledge to each individual patient to develop an individualised care plan without deviating from evidence-based medicine. There is little value in understanding a test result without understanding when to do the test, or the pharmacokinetics of a drug without understanding when to prescribe it. The basic sciences are rigorously tested in the Part 1 exam with a combination of pure and applied science questions. The Part 2 exam focuses on the application of clinical knowledge, so why do candidates who have passed both written papers fail the applied clinical knowledge assessment in the Part 3 exam?

Common pitfalls:

- Patchy knowledge where gaps are exposed by the intense assessment of a ten-minute task.
- A 'scattergun' approach to the task.
- Slavishly following a pathway by failing to understand which are the relevant parts of a guideline to apply to the task.
- Not understanding the significance of co-morbidities in modifying standard care.
- Not listening to a patient's wishes in respect of her care.

Each of the three MRCOG examinations are blueprinted to ensure that every one of them covers the entirety of the core curriculum relevant to that examination. It is self-evident that passing candidates will have ensured they have reviewed the evidence base for each section of the curriculum. The 14 modules of the core curriculum that are assessed in the Part 3 exam are described in more detail in Chapter 3 of this revision guide. The borderline candidate typically has patchy knowledge and may have achieved a bare pass at the Part 2 exam due to luck based on the questions which appeared. The Part 3 exam assesses both comprehensive evidence-based clinical knowledge and the critical thinking to justify the plan that has been made. The Part 3 exam therefore is an assessment of good clinical practice in the real world rather than an assessment of a series of isolated scenarios as each task assesses applied clinical knowledge in the context of assessing other core skills simultaneously.

In order to pass the Part 3 exam you must be able to interpret clinical findings and investigations accurately in order to develop a well-organised management plan. You should be able to justify your plan both in light of the evidence base and the individual patient factors such as age, parity, ethnicity, culture and beliefs. This will include an understanding of the risks and benefits of various management options.

An example of this is the NICE guideline for the management of heavy menstrual bleeding (HMB), which defines a pathway for investigation and subsequent management of HMB. The guideline suggests that the levonorgestrel intrauterine system (LNG-IUS) should be first-line management for HMB. If, however, the scenario is a young woman who wishes to try to conceive in the next 6–12 months, then the LNG-IUS is a very expensive intervention and this woman should be offered more flexible treatment in the form of tranexamic acid and if necessary cyclical progestogens. If on the other hand the scenario is a woman in her late forties who has been sterilised, the competent candidate may be expected to explain to her the benefits of the LNG-IUS in treating HMB, and the potential for it to then be used as part of combined hormone replacement therapy if needed in due course.

This is a very simple example of how to apply a national evidence-based guideline while individualising treatment and being able to justify decision-making in terms of a holistic approach to patient-centred care. The competent candidate will be able to justify why they have taken a modified approach to the guideline. This is very different from ignoring or deviating from the guidance and developing a management plan without reference to the evidence base. It is recognised that not all clinical workplaces will implement the evidence-based guidelines and this may be due to local factors, resources and cultures. Candidates should therefore carefully prepare for the MRCOG by familiarising themselves with these guidelines. When asked to justify a decision or plan in the Part 3 exam, the answer should never be 'because that's the way my consultant does it'; the answer should show a justified application of the relevant guideline.

The previous format of the MRCOG exam did not penalise a candidate with a scattergun approach to answering either the short-answer questions in the written paper or the structured viva stations in the OSCE. Examiners had a checklist of correct answers and candidates could gain marks just by mentioning the answers on the mark sheet, even if their approach was illogical or unstructured. Taking this approach to patient care could result in patients having unnecessary investigations which may incur risks associated with tests or unnecessary costs to the NHS. An important part of evidence-based medicine is to carry out all of the correct tests while understanding which investigations are superfluous.

The Part 3 exam assesses this aspect of applied clinical knowledge and unless your plan for investigation or management demonstrates that you have the critical appraisal skills to formulate a focused and specific plan, you are unlikely to achieve a pass in that task by simply saying anything and everything that comes to mind during the task. The reason for this is that the pressures of exams are similar to the pressures of competing demands on doctors on a busy shift, and the ability to work under pressure while continuing to apply clinical knowledge and principles of patient safety is confirmation of competence and ability to move from core to higher training.

The Part 3 exam will assess your ability to critically appraise differing medical media such as audit reports, scientific papers or clinical guidelines, and then apply this knowledge to the specific scenario in the task. You should be able to analyse the material to devise a plan of investigation, management, treatment or follow-up, and be able to justify your plan to the examiner.

Clinical guidelines are systematically developed statements and the methodology for producing a guideline is specified in the RCOG Clinical Governance Advice Number 1.

The recommendations in all clinical guidelines are classified according to evidence levels and then graded according to the strength of that body of evidence. The guidelines explicitly state that they are not rules to dictate clinical care in every case; rather, they are to be evaluated with reference to individual patient needs. Summaries of the evidence levels and grading system are given at the end of each guideline. The examiner will expect the competent candidate to critically appraise guidance according to evidence levels and be able to justify how they have applied sections of the guidance to the specific task.

Suggestions for Developing Applied Clinical Knowledge Skills

- Do an honest gap analysis of your knowledge and check that you really are familiar with the relevant guidelines for the 14 modules.
- Pick some cases you've recently managed and compare them with the guidelines. Ask yourself the following questions:
  - Did you follow the guidance?
  - Did you have to develop an individualised care plan?
  - Did you request any unnecessary investigations?
  - Could your plan have been more patient-centred?
- Review evidence levels for guidelines.

Conclusions

Miller's skills triangle (Figure 2.1) is a useful representation of how learners develop their skills.

The transition for core to higher training is marked by the transition from 'knowing how' to 'showing how' and 'doing'. The Part 3 exam is firmly based on sound knowledge, but in order to achieve a pass you will need to demonstrate how you apply that knowledge using the five core clinical skills discussed in this chapter. It is essential to critically appraise your own clinical skills and to practise techniques to improve or to avoid common pitfalls so that in nerve-wracking exam conditions you will still demonstrate your strengths. Ultimately these skills will form an essential part of working as a senior, independent clinician.

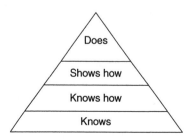

Figure 2.1 Miller's skills triangle.

Additional Resources

Academy of Medical Royal Colleges, Standards for the design of hospital in-patient prescription charts. www.aomrc.org.uk/projects/standards-for-the-design-of-hospital-in-patient-prescription-charts.html

Bayes theorem: Bayes, Thomas (1763) An essay towards solving a problem in the doctrine of chances. *Philosophical Transactions of the Royal Society* 53: 370–418.

Data Protection Act: www.gov.uk/data-protection/the-data-protection-act

GMC (2013; updated April 2014). *Good Medical Practice.* www.gmc-uk.org/static/documents/content/GMP_.pdf

GMC consent: www.gmc-uk.org/Consent___English_1015.pdf_48903482.pdf

Lord Fraser competency: www.nspcc.org.uk/preventing-abuse/child-protection-system/legal-definition-child-rights-law/gillick-competency-fraser-guidelines/n

MBBRACE: www.npeu.ox.ac.uk/mbrrace-uk

Mental Capacity Act: www.nhs.uk/conditions/social-care-and-support-guide/pages/mental-capacity.aspx

Miller, GE (1990). The assessment of clinical skills/competence/performance. *Academic Medicine* 65(7):S63–S67.

MRCOG curriculum: www.rcog.org.uk/en/careers-training/specialty-training-curriculum/core-curriculum

RCOG Clinical Governance Advice No. 1. www.rcog.org.uk/en/guidelines-research-services/guidelines/clinical-governance-advice-1a

3 The Modules of the Curriculum Assessed in the Part 3 Exam

Introduction

The curriculum for the Part 3 exam consists of 14 modules as shown in Table 3.1. These 14 modules are taken from the key clinical areas most suited to assessment by means of a clinical examination of this nature. Table 3.1 links the Part 3 modules to the core curriculum.

Each of the Part 3 modules relates directly to the standards required of an ST5 within the corresponding existing module in the core curriculum. Thus it can be seen that the level of clinical knowledge required to successfully pass the Part 3 exam is no different from the clinical knowledge required to pass the Part 2 exam.

There is, however, a clear difference in the approach to the assessment of knowledge in Part 2, and assessing the application of that knowledge in a clinical setting in the Part 3 exam. As any obstetrician and gynaecologist will know, many patients do not fit a textbook diagnosis and often they will have other co-morbidities, personal issues and beliefs or reasons which mean that standard management is not necessarily appropriate. Within the Part 3 exam, your ability to seek appropriate information from patients,

Table 3.1

	Part 3 module name	Corresponding core curriculum module
1	Teaching	2 (teaching part only)
2	Core surgical skills	5
3	Post-operative care	6
4	Antenatal care	8
5	Maternal medicine	9
6	Management of labour	10
7	Management of delivery	11
8	Postpartum problems (the puerperium)	12
9	Gynaecological problems	13
10	Subfertility	14
11	Sexual and reproductive health	15
12	Early pregnancy care	16
13	Gynaecological oncology	17
14	Urogynaecology and pelvic floor problems	18

communicate effectively with them and your colleagues, and use your clinical knowledge to manage any given clinical situation safely will be tested. The Part 3 exam assessment template (Appendix 1) shows how the five core clinical skills can be applied to each of the 14 modules.

Each Part 3 exam will follow the same format. Each task will be 12 minutes long, consisting of two minutes of reading/preparation time and ten minutes of active examination. The tasks will take one of two broad formats, some with a simulated patient with whom you will interact only, ignoring the examiner, and some with an examiner with whom you will have a structured discussion, rather like a case-based discussion. Do remember that in either type of task you may have one (clinical) examiner, or two (clinical and lay) examiners. If you have two examiners they will both be looking for the same broad information, but the lay examiner will be assessing your skills from a patient's perspective rather than a clinician's.

For each task you will be given a certain amount of material to read in the two minutes you are outside the booth prior to commencing the task. This information will include the types of task you are about to undertake, the domains being assessed and the background to the clinical scenario you are about to face. In writing the exam questions, the question-writing committee spends a considerable amount of time looking at the wording you are given, and removing anything that is unnecessary or might be confusing. It is therefore very important that in the two minutes' preparation time you consider how you might approach the scenario. If there is some information which seems unimportant and unnecessary, have a careful think about it. It is quite likely that it has been put there for a reason and you may need to refer to it later.

Before you start the exam you will be given a pad of paper and a pencil. While you will not be allowed to take these away afterwards, they are yours for making notes or drawing diagrams to help you explain things to simulated patients or examiners if you wish to. Try not to use them for copying down the question during your two minutes outside the booth. All the information on the outside for you to read during the two minutes will also be affixed to the desk in front of you inside the booth for you to refer to if you need to.

How to Approach this Chapter

This chapter contains a section for each of the 14 modules of the Part 3 exam. Each section comprises a brief introduction to the module, an example task (question) followed by examiners' notes from which you can extrapolate some of the key skills that define a competent candidate. Some tasks involve an actor, usually playing a simulated patient, while others will be set as a structured discussion with the examiner.

To gain the most value from this part of the book it is suggested that you initially read the first few paragraphs giving some background to each module, and then review the relevant module in the core curriculum[1] and Part 3 assessment template (Appendix 1).

---

[1] www.rcog.org.uk/en/careers-training/specialty-training-curriculum/core-curriculum/

For a simulated patient task you should read the simulated patient's instructions carefully so that you understand the scenario they have been asked to perform. When you are comfortable with the scenario you should spend two minutes reading the candidate's instructions and considering your approach to answering the task. Then, using a timer, spend ten minutes attempting the task either by writing down or discussing with your exam buddy which skills and knowledge you would demonstrate in each of the domains being assessed. When the ten minutes have elapsed, read through the examiner's notes of how a competent candidate would be expected to approach the task.

In the case of a structured conversation you will be told how many examiner's questions have been included. For the purposes of your revision, assume the ten minutes will be divided equally between each of them. Either ask your exam buddy to ask each question in turn, or cover them up and write down your answers for each one.

As you work your way through each module you will notice that some of the example tasks could also be used to assess other modules. For example, the task on teaching consent used to assess module 1 (teaching) could, with a slightly different emphasis, be used to assess module 2 (core surgical skills). When you are comfortable with the example tasks presented within each module, read through them again and write down which other modules each one could possibly be used to assess. Then work on your own or with your exam buddy to see how you might change your answers in order to demonstrate your knowledge and skill from this different viewpoint.

Module 1: Teaching

The Part 3 exam sits as a waypoint at the end of core training. An ST5 passing the examination and obtaining the MRCOG will be entering the final phases of training before becoming a consultant, and as such will, by definition, already have the responsibility of teaching the next generation of trainees in obstetrics and gynaecology. It is therefore essential that they understand not only the principles of adult learning, but also the best ways to impart that knowledge and ensure that the learner has understood what they have been taught and is able to assimilate it and progress in their own training.

This module requires you to understand all aspects of teaching, including the teaching of a practical skill, preparation of a teaching session and the use of audio-visual aids and mannequins. You should have the necessary skills to ensure that more junior trainees fully understand the subject matter of the teaching session in order to ensure patient safety going forwards.

While this module clearly places an emphasis on communication with colleagues, it will also give you the opportunity to demonstrate your abilities in particular aspects of patient safety and applied clinical knowledge. Remember that sometimes patients and their families also need educating on their condition or management, so depending on the scenario that is used in the task, you may need to demonstrate communication with patients and families, or information gathering from an unqualified learner. An example task is given below.

Candidate's Instructions

This is a simulated trainee task assessing the following domains:

- *communication with patients*
- *communication with colleagues*
- *applied clinical knowledge*
- *patient safety.*

You are an ST5, and a junior trainee (second foundation year) has recently joined your department. The trainee will be required to take consent for elective caesarean sections. You are about to carry out a caesarean section for a breech presentation and have noticed that the consent form for this patient has already been filled in by this trainee.

You have ten minutes in which you should:

- *review the consent form with the junior doctor and provide feedback*
- *explain the principles of obtaining valid consent*
- *support the trainee in their ongoing education*

Patient identifier/label	Name: Samantha Brown DOB: 06/09/1986

Name of proposed procedure or course of treatment (include brief explanation if medical term not clear) ...... LSCS ....

Statement of health professional (to be filled in by health professional with appropriate knowledge of proposed procedure, as specified in consent policy)

I have explained the procedure to the patient. In particular, I have explained:

The intended benefits ... Deliver a baby safely ....
...... Through a cut in the abdomen and uterus

Serious or frequently occurring risks ... Haemorrhage, blood clots (1%)
... infection, injury to bladder, bowels (low risk)
... Hysterectomy and cut to baby skin (rare)
Any extra procedures which may become necessary during the procedure

[✓] blood transfusion...

[ ] other procedure (please specify) ....
....

I have also discussed what the procedure is likely to involve, the benefits and risks of any available alternative treatments (including no treatment) and any particular concerns of this patient.

[ ] The following leaflet/tape has been provided ....

This procedure will involve:

[✓] general and/or regional anaesthesia   [ ] local anaesthesia   [ ] sedation

Signed:..   Date .. .. 5/4/16 ......
Name (PRINT) ... Sam Lewis ...   Job title ... ST1 O+G ....

Contact details (if patient wishes to discuss options later) Mrs. Brown Secretary
labour Ward   extension 4132   extension 4605
Statement of Interpreter (where appropriate)

not required

I have interpreted the information above to the patient to the best of my ability and in a way in which I believe s/he can understand.

Signed ....   Date ....
Name (PRINT) ....

Top copy accepted by patient (yes)/no (please ring)

2

Figure 3.1

Simulated Trainee's Instructions

You are a junior trainee in obstetrics one year after qualification (FY2) who has just joined the department on rotation. As part of your duties, you will have to take consent for elective caesarean sections. The midwives asked you to obtain consent from a woman booked to have an elective caesarean section because the baby is in breech presentation, which you have done based on what you can remember from your medical school days.

You always did well at medical school, but there was not much teaching about taking consent during your obstetric module.

You are a self-confident individual and not always good at taking advice from colleagues unless you find what they say convincing.

If not covered by the candidate, you could ask the following questions:

- *Do I need to mention the risks that are really rare?*
- *How could I be expected to fit everything in the form?*
- *If I had included all the risks, wouldn't the patient have refused the procedure?*

The candidate should:

- *highlight the good points in the way consent was documented*
- *explain the principles of obtaining valid consent*
- *outline and correct mistakes in the consent*
- *encourage reflection and self-directed learning*

Notes on Your Approach to the Task

Examiner's Notes

This question provides an opportunity to examine both communication with colleagues and communication with patients. In communicating with patients, a competent candidate would ensure that the consent form contains information written in such a way that a non-medically qualified patient would be able to understand it. Abbreviations should be avoided, as should medical jargon. The writing should be clear and legible.

Equally, in testing communication with colleagues, the competent candidate will first commend the trainee on what they have done well, including the legibility of their writing and the intended benefits. They will provide constructive feedback on how the trainee can improve their approach to consent by understanding the benefits and risk of the procedure and how they should be communicated to the patient. The competent candidate will ensure the junior trainee has understood the implications of what they have been taught, has been able to assimilate it and can repeat when asked the salient points to ensure the learning has been embedded. Of key importance in giving feedback is that it should be done objectively and without undermining the junior trainee.

When looking at information gathering, the competent candidate will first of all identify what the junior trainee understands, what their concerns are and then ensure within the ten minutes that they address these in a manner appropriate to their learning.

The competent candidate will demonstrate their applied clinical knowledge by explaining the principles of obtaining valid consent, including that it must be voluntary and informed, and the person consenting must have the capacity to make the decision. Equally it should be taken by someone who can either undertake the procedure or who has been trained to take consent for that particular procedure. A key assessment of communication with patients will therefore be to explain to the simulated trainee that they should not have taken the consent without prior training, but to do so without undermining them.

In demonstrating patient safety, the competent candidate will ensure the trainee has an accurate understanding of the risks of a caesarean section, correcting the inaccuracies on the form. They will then point the trainee to other resources such as hospital policies, RCOG guidelines, the GMC or the Medical Defence Organisations to consolidate their learning from this brief teaching session.

Reflection on the Task

Review the notes you made before reading the examiner's notes. Did you remember the principles of informed consent, patient safety and giving formative feedback to a junior colleague to ensure learning?

- Legible writing avoiding abbreviations
- Documenting risks and alternatives to operation
- Assessment of mental capacity
- Not taking consent if unable to discuss the procedure and alternatives
- Principles of feedback
- Supportive approach to going beyond training – patient safety

Module 2: Core Surgical Skills

This module covers surgical procedures in an obstetric and gynaecological context and expects a clear understanding of pre-operative assessment, intra-operative procedures and complications. Obviously some tasks used in this module could also be used to assess module 3, post-operative care.

While the majority of surgical training and surgical skills will be assessed through workplace-based assessments in the operating theatre, particularly through formative and summative OSATS, there is an opportunity and an expectation within the Part 3 exam for your knowledge of a number of aspects pertaining more broadly to general surgical skills, such as applied anatomy and the use and design of certain instruments, to be tested. While you may not be able to manage the more major intra-operative complications, there is an expectation that you will be able to identify them and know the principles of their management.

It is important to realise that this module does not solely test operative experience and knowledge, but as surgical safety is of primary importance throughout obstetrics and gynaecology the tasks used to assess you in this module will not only have a major emphasis on the principles of safe surgery, but also the clinical governance aspects of the identification of poor outcomes and their management. Within this, your ability to coordinate and manage an operating list, and use the broader operating theatre staff to get the most out of them as a team, could also be assessed. An example task is given below.

Candidate's Instructions

This structured discussion assesses:

- *communication with colleagues*
- *communication with patients*
- *applied clinical knowledge*
- *patient safety.*

You are an ST5 undertaking an elective caesarean section. The consultant is dictating letters in the theatre office and you are assisted by a year-two foundation doctor.

The patient has a BMI of 31. Her past obstetric history includes two caesarean sections, the first for a breech presentation and the second for failure to progress in labour.

You open the abdomen through a transverse lower abdominal incision using the previous scar. As you reflect the bladder you notice some clear fluid and realise that the bladder has accidentally been opened.

You have ten minutes to have a structured conversation with the examiner, who has four questions they can use to discuss with you the subsequent management of this patient.

Examiner's Instructions

Familiarise yourself with the candidate's instructions.

Use the following four questions as a guide to conduct a structured discussion with the candidate:

- *What immediate action would you take?*
- *What is your approach to completion of the operation?*
- *What is your post-operative management plan?*
- *What issues would you discuss with the patient post-operatively?*

Notes on Your Approach to the Task

Examiner's Notes

The competent candidate will first and foremost realise that in this situation they have two patients to consider. The initial key aspect of patient safety will be that, as an ST5, the candidate is unlikely to be competent at repairing the damaged bladder and so will have to seek help. This should be done immediately by clearly informing the anaesthetist and scrub nurse, and calling the consultant to theatre to help assess the site and extent of the bladder injury. The consultant can then decide whether urological assistance is required. In the meantime, the competent candidate will realise they cannot prejudice the condition of the fetus due to the bladder injury; therefore, as long as they can enter the lower segment of the uterus without further damaging the bladder in order to deliver the baby safely, they should continue to do so.

While a competent candidate cannot be expected to be able to repair a bladder injury unsupervised, by applying their clinical knowledge they should have an understanding of the principles of such a repair and its management, such as using a two-layer approach with an absorbable suture, and considering a peritoneal drain to ensure there is no extravasation of urine through the repair. In addition, they should be able to ensure the patient is safe post-operatively with an indwelling Foley catheter and prophylactic antibiotics. The competent candidate will have a clear and coherent plan for the patient, including good-quality documentation, leaving the catheter for around seven days, with clear instructions to the nursing staff to avoid it blocking, and what to do if it does. A competent candidate will also realise that this patient is likely to be less mobile post-operatively as a result of the catheter and therefore will consider extending the duration of her thromboprophylaxis.

The communication aspects of this task are two-fold. Communication with colleagues has already been discussed above, both in calling for help and the post-operative management plan. The competent candidate's approach to communication with the patient will, however, be very important. The competent candidate will realise that as this is an elective caesarean section there is every possibility that the woman would be awake, and so will hear the initial conversations with colleagues. They will therefore ensure the patient is not unduly frightened during the procedure, and explain to the woman and her partner immediately afterwards both what has happened and why, and how this will affect her post-operative recovery. They will also be reassuring that the patient is unlikely to suffer any long-term ill-effects.

Reflection on the Task

Review the notes that you made before reading the examiner's notes. Did you remember the principles of safe surgery, calling for help and making a reasoned plan? Did you consider the clinical governance issues and the need to explain what happened to the patient (duty of candour)?

- Inform theatre team
- Call for help
- If you can do so, safely deliver the baby while help is on the way
- Explain to the patient
- Deal surgically with the bladder injury
- Make a post-operative management plan
- Complete an incident report form.

Module 3: Post-Operative Care

Good post-operative care following all surgical procedures is essential in both obstetrics and gynaecology. The rationale behind this module is to ensure that you understand the physiological and psychological principles needed to ensure every patient makes a safe and effective recovery following their procedure. There is also a specific expectation within the core curriculum that an ST5 will be able to debrief patients following most complications.

As a competent ST5 you should be able to manage a patient's care from the initial procedure through to discharge and beyond. This includes not only fluid and catheter management, analgesia and wound management, but also the ability to identify complications and explain them to patients and their families in a way they can understand. You should request appropriate investigations which you can justify, but not undertake unnecessary tests. You should be able to explain post-operative recovery after the patient has been discharged from hospital, including return to work. There is much evidence that for most patients, short hospital stays are beneficial to both the patient and the organisation, so you should ensure you manage your patients in such a way as to keep them safe but also have resources for all patients, as given in the example below.

Candidate's Instructions

This task uses a structured discussion to assess:

- *communication with colleagues*
- *communication with patients*
- *applied clinical knowledge*
- *patient safety.*

   You are an ST5 and have been asked to update the patient-information leaflet entitled 'Coming to Hospital for Abdominal Hysterectomy' to incorporate 'Enhanced Recovery'. Your consultant has asked you to discuss your views with him.

   You have ten minutes in which you should:

- *explain the principles and benefits of the Enhanced Recovery Programme*
- *suggest how the leaflet should be changed to fit with the principles of enhanced recovery*

Existing Patient Information Leaflet

Coming to Hospital for Abdominal Hysterectomy

This leaflet is to give you a guide on what to expect when coming into the gynaecology unit. If you require more information about any aspect, please do not hesitate to ask the staff.

Before Admission
You will be seen by a nurse in a pre-operative clinic a week before your operation, who will assess you and will carry out routine tests. You may need to meet the anaesthetist to discuss issues relevant to your anaesthetic. Please bring with you any medications you are taking. Let us know about any allergies as we will be giving antibiotics during your operation.

Admission to Hospital
You will come into hospital the day before your surgery. You will need an enema to empty your bowels the night before your operation. You will then stop eating and drinking from midnight and we will ask you to wear tight-fitting stockings to prevent blood clots from developing in your veins.

After Your Operation
When you come back from theatre you will have a needle in your arm for intravenous fluids, a tube to drain your bladder (catheter) and a small drain near your wound for any collected blood. These are likely to be removed after a day or two, but occasionally may need to remain for longer. You must not eat or drink until the medical staff tell you that it is safe to do so, usually after your bowel returns to normal. You will be given plenty of painkillers.

The Days After Your Operation
You will be encouraged to start slowly mobilising when you feel comfortable. You will be given an injection to prevent blood clots developing in your veins. We will ensure you are able to pass urine after the catheter is removed, but if you have difficulties it may need to be re-inserted.

Leaving Hospital
Most women will be able to leave hospital about five days after the operation, but this may vary. Before you go home we will ensure that you are pain-free and your bowels have opened.

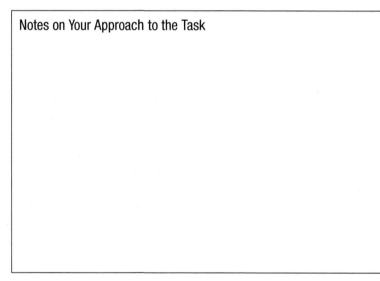

Examiner's Notes

It can be seen that this task is based on an example of a patient leaflet which is used to support a case-based discussion with the examiner around care following an abdominal hysterectomy and the candidate's understanding of enhanced recovery.

In this task, first and foremost the competent candidate will be tested on their ability to discuss with the examiner, using evidence, how the leaflet can be improved and in doing so their communication skills with both patients and colleagues will be assessed.

The competent candidate will be able to explain to the examiner how and why enhanced recovery facilitates speedier recovery and earlier discharge for the patient, and the advantages of this to both the patient and to the hospital. They will be aware it is a generic model of care designed to facilitate faster recovery following elective surgery, and is not confined to gynaecology, the aim being to promote earlier hospital discharge and a faster return to normal activities for the patient.

When describing the components of the enhanced recovery programme, the competent candidate will communicate in a logical fashion – for example, beginning with pre-operative care, then intra-operative care, followed by post-operative care. They should also be able to clearly describe the advantages for patients in terms of quicker return to normal activities and improved patient satisfaction.

This task also examines communication with patients in a written form, as the competent candidate will be able to demonstrate to the examiner the substitution of technical terms within the leaflet for simple lay terms that the patient and her family will understand. They will clearly demonstrate both the general rationale behind giving written rather than verbal information, as well as any specific issues relating to hysterectomy. They should explain that the provision of a leaflet alone does not constitute imparting information and that even the best-written leaflets may require explanation and possible translation, depending on the patient with whom they are dealing. They should also demonstrate the advantages of including contact telephone numbers to allow the patient access to clinical (often nursing) support, but also the use of structured proactive telephone follow-up to ensure the patient remains safe and well following discharge.

From a patient safety perspective, the competent candidate will understand the need for pre-operative optimisation of patients, both from the point of view of any long-term conditions she may have (such as high blood pressure) as well as physiological optimisation such as losing weight, exercise and stopping smoking. They will understand that, while enhanced recovery delivers efficient admission to hospital prior to a procedure along with systems to support prompt return to normal physiological processes, where necessary there will be clear processes in place to ensure that if a patient deviates from the prescribed path there is a suitable index of suspicion to ensure that post-operative complications are fully and appropriately managed. In addition, the shorter period of immobility and dehydration should be discussed as a means of further reducing the risk of venous thrombosis.

Finally, the competent candidate will demonstrate knowledgeable application of their clinical understanding by underpinning the conversation with examples of the components of enhanced recovery throughout the patient journey. They should ensure that throughout the conversation with the examiner they discuss appropriate care in relation to an abdominal hysterectomy and do not drift into other procedures such as vaginal or laparoscopic hysterectomy. The competent candidate should also demonstrate the limitations of their knowledge by not discussing in any significant detail anaesthesia, or elements of nursing or physiotherapy care, which are outside the MRCOG curriculum.

Reflection on the Task

Review the notes you made before reading the examiner's notes. Did you remember the four domains being assessed in this task and make relevant notes for each one? In communicating with colleagues did you appreciate the need to give feedback on the leaflet by adhering to the general principles of feedback by commenting on both what was good as well as what could be improved?

- Leaflet – constructive comments, good and bad
- Enhanced recovery – process and benefits for the patient
- Logical approach
- Use of language/jargon
- Limitations of giving leaflets rather than discussion.

Module 4: Antenatal Care

Well-planned and delivered antenatal care is fundamental to good obstetric outcomes. As an ST5 you should not only understand the principles behind routine midwifery care in the low-risk woman, but also how to identify a range of risk factors and produce an individualised management plan to suit the needs of a range of obstetric patients. In addition you should be able to then review each individual plan, and modify it as necessary in response to changing or additional risks that may occur throughout the antenatal period.

Communication with women and their families is key to good antenatal care, so you will be expected to be very clear when sharing results of investigations, be they good or bad, and ensuring women are fully informed of any management plan you may suggest or any decisions they may have to make. Communication with colleagues at all levels from community settings (midwives and general practitioners) to senior consultants should demonstrate that you have identified any risks, and if possible ensured that these can be mitigated and managed appropriately, to ultimately maximise the chances of a safe and successful birth for mother and baby.

A typical task is shown below.

Candidate's Instructions (1)

This is a simulated patient task assessing:

- *communication with patients*
- *information gathering*
- *patient safety*
- *applied clinical knowledge.*

You are an ST5 working in a district general hospital. You are about to see Mrs Lambert, who has been sent to the antenatal clinic because she seems to have a small baby. An ultrasound scan has already been carried out. The result is shown on the next sheet.

You have ten minutes in which you should:

- *obtain a relevant history*
- *explain the scan result*
- *establish and answer the patient's concerns*
- *outline and justify a management plan*

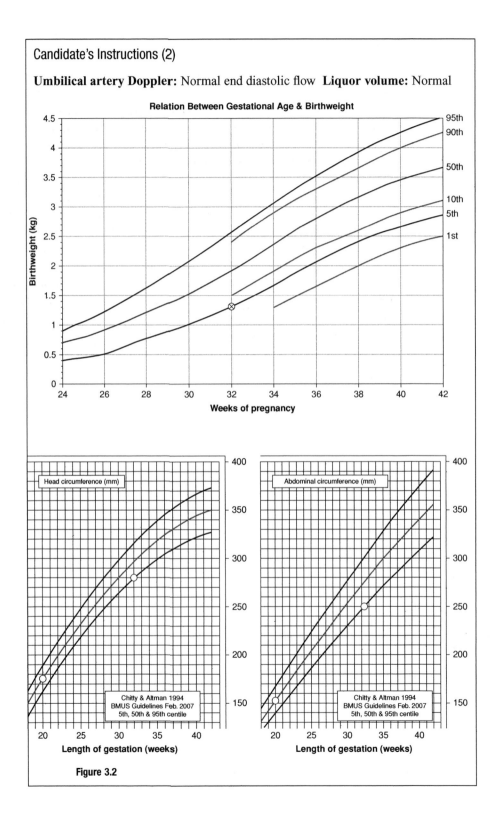

Candidate's Instructions (2)

Umbilical artery Doppler: Normal end diastolic flow **Liquor volume:** Normal

Figure 3.2

Simulated Patient's Instructions

You are Mrs Carolyn Lambert, a 36-year-old actress. You have been in a stable relationship with Clark, a 38-year-old actor, for five years. You are both in good health, only occasionally drink alcohol and you smoke ten cigarettes each day. You have always attended a gym three times per week and have continued to do so while you have been pregnant. Your fitness is very important to you and you intend to keep exercising and working until the end of the pregnancy.

This is your first pregnancy and you are 32 weeks pregnant. A scan at the beginning of your pregnancy confirmed your dates to be correct. A further scan at 20 weeks showed no abnormalities in your baby, which was growing normally. You had all the usual screening tests carried out and they were also reported as normal. You have recently moved to the area so all these tests were done at your previous hospital. The baby is active.

You are attending the antenatal clinic because your community midwife thinks your baby is small. You had a scan yesterday but do not know the result. You are not worried about the situation as you think your baby is fine and you are too busy for a lot of extra visits to the antenatal clinic.

If not covered by the candidate, you could ask the following questions:

- *What does the scan show?*
- *Is my baby normal?*
- *Is my baby small?*
- *Why is my baby small?*
- *What happens now?*
- *What might happen until I am due?*

Notes on Your Approach to the Task

Examiner's Notes

In order to be able to answer the patient's questions, the competent candidate will take a brief directed history, in particular to ascertain the results of any previous investigations or scans, but also any risk factors for growth restriction such as smoking or exercise. With only ten minutes to complete the task, the competent candidate will realise that a full history cannot be completed and so will confine themselves to questions that will aid in their diagnosis and management of this patient.

At all times, the competent candidate's communication with the patient will need to be objective and not judgemental, yet firm when discussing issues such as smoking. The first point to establish will be what the patient already understands. When explaining the implications of the scan result, and the subsequent management plan, the good candidate will discuss empathetically the possible scenarios and decisions that the woman may have to take depending on the results of subsequent serial scans.

The competent candidate's explanation of the scan will support the examiner's assessment of them in the domain of applied clinical knowledge. They should explain that all measurements are on the 5th centile, and while this may be normal, it is below the 10th centile, which has the best sensitivity and specificity for detecting growth restriction. Therefore we cannot be certain as to whether it is a concern or not, until serial growth scans have shown a normal growth velocity. On the positive side, the competent candidate will provide some reassurance to the mother from the normal Doppler result.

Within this task it is the baby that is at the greatest risk. The competent candidate will demonstrate a clear plan to observe the baby by umbilical artery Doppler and ultrasound estimation of fetal weight, size and liquor volume, but will acknowledge that the plan may need to be modified depending on the results to ensure patient safety. They will explain two clear options, depending on the outcomes of the ultrasound scans. If the scans remain normal the competent candidate should offer delivery at around 37 weeks; however, if the fetal growth becomes static, delivery might need to be earlier in which case the woman may need steroids for fetal lung maturation. The competent candidate will ensure that a fetal medicine specialist is consulted as the scanning techniques are beyond the required competencies expected of an ST5.

Reflection on the Task

Review the notes you made before reading the examiner's notes. Did you develop an approach that covered all four domains being assessed?

- Focused history considering time management
- Clear explanation of the scan findings
- Justification of the management plan
- Logical approach to the plan.

Module 5: Maternal Medicine

The maternal medicine module offers the opportunity to assess you against all five domains across a wide range of clinical situations. Within the core curriculum you will see that you are expected to understand the aetiology and pathophysiology of maternal diseases in almost every organ system of the body, but also under direct supervision be able to diagnose and manage them. You should be able to manage many of the more common diseases, such as hypertension, asthma and haemoglobinopathy, to name but a few, largely independently through your experience. With less common conditions you should be able to demonstrate a sensible initial approach to management, followed by clear communication with an appropriate specialist colleague.

The tasks within this module can be used to demonstrate your abilities in managing patients from preconception throughout antenatal care and labour to the puerperium. The tasks can cover both common or rare medical or psychiatric conditions as well as social issues such as domestic violence. In addition a task can be set to test your ability to manage the effect of medical conditions or their treatment on the pregnant mother or the fetus, or alternatively the effect of being pregnant on the medical condition.

A typical task is shown below.

Candidate's Instructions

This is a simulated patient task assessing:

- *communication with patients*
- *information gathering*
- *patient safety*
- *applied clinical knowledge.*

    You are an ST5 working in the clinic. You are about to see Martha Macdonald. The referral letter from her general practitioner is as follows:

Windy Ridge Surgery
Cliff Top Road
Strathclyde
ST5 5BB

Dear Obstetrician,

Re: Martha McDonald

Please could you see Ms Martha McDonald who is aged 33. She was diagnosed with asthma at the age of 17 years. For the last six years she has been hospitalised at least once a year with acute severe attacks.

    She has a daughter, born four years ago, at 31 weeks of gestation by caesarean section because of a significant deterioration in Ms McDonald's respiratory function. The baby was small for dates. She smokes 5–10 cigarettes a day. Her BMI is 31 and she is trying to lose weight.

    She has a new partner and would like to have a baby with him, but is concerned about the risks. She wishes to receive more information about possible complications and whether her medication is safe for pregnancy.

    Her current medications are: prednisolone 40 mg daily, budesonide (Symbicort®) inhaler, ipratropium bromide (Atrovent®) nebulisers, montelukast (Singulair®) 10 mg daily, terbutaline (Bricanyl®), omeprazole 20 mg daily

Yours sincerely,

Dr Marcus Bloomhead FRCGP

You have ten minutes in which you should:

- *advise on the potential risks/complications of another pregnancy*
- *outline a specific management plan for before and during pregnancy*
- *answer any questions the patient may ask*

Simulated Patient's Instructions

You are Martha McDonald, a 33-year-old part-time secretary. You were diagnosed with asthma at the age of 17 years. Initially the condition was reasonably mild and stable. However, for the last six years the asthma attacks have been more severe and frequent. You have been in hospital at least once per year due to a sudden attack and you now need much more medication to help your breathing.

You have had one previous pregnancy four years ago during which your asthma deteriorated and you were in hospital from about 26 weeks of pregnancy. You were delivered at 31 weeks by caesarean section because of concerns about your deteriorating breathlessness. After delivery, you remember spending several days in the intensive care unit because of concerns about your asthma and breathing. Your daughter weighed less than 1 kg and she spent ten weeks in the special care baby unit. It took you quite a long time to get back to normal after the delivery.

You smoke 5–10 cigarettes each day. You know this is inadvisable but you cannot stop. You have put some weight on since the birth but have been attending Weight Watchers and are trying to lose weight.

You have a new partner and you would like to have a baby with him, but you are worried about the risks, especially as you were so ill during the last pregnancy. You would like information about possible complications for you and your baby because of your asthma, your medication and your previous caesarean section. The medication you are currently taking seems to suit you and you feel that your asthma is under reasonable control at the moment.

If not covered by the candidate, you could ask the following questions:

- *Will my asthma get worse in pregnancy again? Could I die?*
- *Will the medicine I take harm the baby?*
- *Will I need another caesarean section?*
- *If asked, say you have not been referred to a stop-smoking service or tried nicotine replacement.*

Notes on Your Approach to the Task

Examiner's Notes

First and foremost, the competent candidate will gather information quickly to establish how brittle this woman's asthma is, and what happened during her first pregnancy, both in terms of her antenatal admission and her post-operative recovery. They will also need to enquire how her current condition compares to her condition before her first pregnancy. The competent candidate will enquire about smoking, and emphasise the need to provide support to help her stop, both for her general health as well as to maximise her chances of a successful pregnancy.

The competent candidate will demonstrate separately three aspects of their applied clinical knowledge.

First, they will describe the maternal risks such as a significant risk of deterioration which could be life threatening, or prolonged separation from her daughter due to hospitalisation.

Second, they will discuss risks to the baby, particularly perinatal mortality or morbidity due to premature delivery. They should be reassuring about prednisolone, which does not cause fetal abnormalities, but be aware that there is limited safety data on montelukast so will need to consult with the local drug information service. Other risks to the fetus will include growth restriction and adrenal suppression due to high-dose steroids, both of which will be clearly addressed by the competent candidate.

Finally, they should offer a possible management plan whereby they optimise asthma control before conception and use a reliable method of contraception until Ms McDonald's condition has been optimised. They should refer her to a smoking cessation service and suggest she sees her GP for nicotine replacement. The competent candidate will then offer reassurance that once she is pregnant she will have access to multidisciplinary care, prompt treatment of any asthma attack and that the most appropriate method of delivery will need to be decided when there is a clearer understanding of the clinical situation she is facing at the time.

Untreated or poorly managed, this could be a life-threatening situation for this woman. The competent candidate will therefore communicate the risks to both the mother and the baby in an objective but sympathetic manner. They will portray the risks in a realistic fashion and allow the patient to make an informed choice about whether she has another baby or not. They should not use medical terms, but may pull on her experience from her first pregnancy and her subsequent progress to illustrate the risks.

Finally, this task will assess patient safety from both the perspective of the mother and the baby. The risks to the mother will not just relate to the asthma itself, but also to the treatment in the form of the risks of thrombosis due to prolonged hospitalisation and the risk of gestational diabetes as a result of steroid administration. The risks of prematurity may be significant to the fetus, but the competent candidate will explain that in extreme circumstances it may even be necessary to make decisions between the life of the mother or the baby.

Reflection on the Task

Review the notes you made before reading the examiner's notes. It's really important to realise this is a pre-conception counselling session and the simulated patient could choose to become pregnant or avoid pregnancy based on your advice.

- Use a non-judgemental approach to sensitive issues – smoking and BMI
- Discuss potentially life-threatening asthmas without unduly scaring the patient
- Use negotiation skills
- Consider safety in respect of prescribing in pregnancy
- Explain the multidisciplinary approach.

Module 6: Management of Labour

A clear understanding of the management of both normal and abnormal labour is at the very heart of the MRCOG examination. While the majority of procedures associated with labour will be assessed using summative and formative workplace-based assessments, including non-technical skills such as coordinating a delivery suite, these skills can also be objectively assessed through this module of the Part 3 exam.

The breadth of this module allows all five domains to be tested. Tasks can be set under applied clinical knowledge that ensure the candidate can manage individual women and their deliveries, complications of labour, breaking bad news and the management of the delivery suite as a whole.

Safety is paramount on the delivery suite, and you can expect some aspect of the ability to care for both women and their babies safely to be tested in every exam. One of the key aspects of patient safety on the delivery suite is the handover, both at the beginning and end of each shift, as well as between professionals, making communication with colleagues another important domain within this module.

At the centre of every birth are the woman and her partner. They need to be kept informed of progress and events throughout the delivery, and whether things go well or not, your ability to communicate clearly and succinctly with women at a time of extreme emotion is the backbone of good obstetric care.

As you will see from the typical task below, not every scenario that relates to labour and delivery will need to be set on the delivery suite.

Candidate's Instructions

This is a simulated patient task assessing:

- *communication with patients*
- *information gathering*
- *patient safety*
- *applied clinical knowledge.*

   You are an ST5 and have been asked to help at the antenatal clinic because the consultant has been called away at short notice. The patient you are about to see is a 32-year-old scientist who has been referred by her general practitioner for management advice. The referral letter is shown below.

Windy Bridge Surgery
530 London Road
Thornton Heath
Croydon
CR7 7YE

Dear Mr Krest

Re: Mary Goodnight

I will be grateful if you would arrange to see Mrs Goodnight at your antenatal clinic. She has just moved to the area and is currently 36 weeks pregnant. When she delivered two years ago she had a fourth-degree tear. She would like to discuss her mode of delivery in this pregnancy.

Yours sincerely

Abdul

Dr Abdul Mohammed, MRCGP

   You have ten minutes in which you should:

- *obtain a detailed history*
- *offer and justify a management plan*
- *answer any questions the patient may have*

Simulated Patient's Instructions

You are Mrs Mary Goodnight, a 32-year-old scientist with a two-year-old daughter. You are in good health, do not smoke and only occasionally drink alcohol. You are not taking any medication and have no allergies. You are married to Ian, a 35-year-old import/export manager. You have just moved into this area.

You are currently 36 weeks pregnant, and you have been referred to the antenatal clinic as you want to discuss how you are going to deliver in this pregnancy. This pregnancy has been entirely normal and you are planning to have at least four children.

You had a bad experience with your first labour. You were induced with three pessaries before your waters were broken. You then went into labour very quickly. You were looked after by a student midwife as the delivery suite was short-staffed, and she seemed to be running between several rooms. No one believed that you were labouring so quickly so you were given an injection of pethidine that made you feel very drowsy for about an hour. You then remember you were told very sharply that you had to push as your daughter was in distress and you had to get her out in two pushes. She was born using suction (ventouse) and weighed 3.2 kg. You were cut, but also suffered a nasty tear to your anus. You were rushed to theatre to have everything stitched. Your daughter has not had any problems.

You recovered well from your tear but received very poor aftercare and no follow-up. You think they told you that you had a fourth-degree tear but should be able to have a normal birth next time. You were never sent an appointment to attend a postnatal clinic to discuss this, so are very keen to have a caesarean section to avoid any possibility of another tear, and because the whole experience was so frightening last time.

Once everything settled after the birth you have not had any bowel or urinary problems. You do not leak flatus (wind).

If not covered by the candidate, you could ask the following questions:

- *Can I have a caesarean section?*
- *Why have I been advised to have a vaginal birth?*
- *If I have a vaginal birth, how can you reduce the chance of me tearing again?*

Notes on Your Approach to the Task

Examiner's Notes

Communication with patients will be one of the key areas this task assesses, but equally one that the competent candidate should excel at, as this type of conversation will be taking place every week in every obstetric unit. Counselling a patient that their preferred mode of delivery may not be the most appropriate for them, and ensuring that it is done in an objective non-directional manner is a skill essential to every obstetrician. The competent candidate will listen to her concerns and explain, using their obstetric knowledge and experience, what the woman's options are in clear and plain language that will allow her to make an informed choice about how she would like to have this baby.

In order to have an objective conversation the competent candidate will take a brief history to obtain details of the previous delivery and tear, as well as the post-operative recovery and support (or not) that was provided. It is also important to ascertain her current symptoms, her preferred method of delivery and the reasons behind it, including her long-term plans for further children.

To demonstrate their applied clinical knowledge, the competent candidate will propose a clearly reasoned management plan to the woman which takes into account evidence-based advice, but also offers an element of compromise, reassurance and negotiation with the woman in order to build her confidence. By explaining that vaginal delivery is a very reasonable option as she has no residual bowel symptoms and there is a low chance of needing instrumental delivery again, the woman's fears and misconceptions may be allayed. However, the competent candidate will take into account her wishes for four children and balance the discussion of the risks of vaginal delivery with both the positive benefits of caesarean section on the pelvic floor and the risks of subsequent caesareans.

To ensure the woman's safety, the competent candidate will include in their counselling that there is no evidence to suggest use of prophylactic episiotomy. They will explain the risks of repeat caesarean clearly and objectively, including intra-operative risks such as bowel or bladder adhesions or a morbidly adherent placenta. They will acknowledge the patient's right to choose the mode of delivery, explaining that it is the doctor's job to ensure the woman has all the information she needs to make an informed choice. Finally, to ensure that they have all the information they need to help this woman, the competent candidate will offer to obtain details from the previous hospital to be certain that there were no other issues which might affect this delivery.

Reflection on the Task

Review the notes that you made before reading the examiner's notes. Time management is key to this task. The clear instruction to take a detailed history should be interpreted as a very focused detailed history. The candidate who doesn't discover the patient's plans for four children will miss a key element of decision-making and safety.

- Giving both pros and cons of vaginal and caesarean delivery is essential.
- The woman should be able to use information to make her own choice rather than be told what to do.
- Negotiation and compromise are key skills being tested.
- Practise agreeing a plan rather than deciding for the patient.

Module 7: Management of Delivery

This module follows directly from the previous one (management of labour), but while there may be some apparent overlaps, if you look at the Part 3 clinical assessment template (Appendix 1) you will clearly see the differences. It should be obvious that, having these two modules in any given sitting of the exam, there will be a significant emphasis on situations that might be encountered in acute obstetric practice. In addition, this is a module with some very practical aspects so it lends itself to being assessed alongside both teaching (module 1) as well as surgical care (modules 2 and 3).

Module 7 covers both the practical aspects of normal and assisted delivery, be it vaginal or abdominal, as well as the decision-making around the urgency and most appropriate time and place to deliver a woman.

Communication will feature prominently in the assessment of this module, as it is key to safe management of patients on any delivery suite. Equally, as patient expectations are not always achievable and perfect outcomes cannot be guaranteed, how you negotiate with patients will be very important.

A typical task dealing with delivery is shown below.

Candidate's Instructions

This task is a four-part structured discussion covering:

- *applied clinical knowledge*
- *patient safety*
- *communication with colleagues.*

You are the ST5 on call for labour ward admissions. You are asked to attend Rachael Brown, who has been admitted with a 12-hour history of colicky lower abdominal pain which is increasing in frequency. She is 31 weeks into her first pregnancy according to a dating ultrasound scan at 12 weeks. It is a singleton pregnancy with a cephalic presentation and her symphyseal fundal height is 32 cm. The uterus is not tender but there is tenderness in the right renal angle. There are no signs of previous surgery.

She has had no bleeding or fluid loss from the vagina. There is no history of urinary frequency, haematuria or dysuria. Fetal movements have not changed.

Her blood group is O Rhesus positive. The pregnancy has been uneventful to date.

You have ten minutes in which you should discuss the diagnosis and management of this clinical scenario with the examiner. The examiner has four questions around which to structure the discussion.

Examiner's Instructions

You should divide the task equally between the four statements below within the ten minutes. At each stage you should tell the candidate the additional information then begin the discussion by covering the following points:

- *Justify any additional clinical examination that you would like to perform.*
- *Uterine contractions are occurring every ten minutes and are moderate in strength. On vaginal examination the cervix is fully effaced and 1 cm dilated. What is your differential diagnosis and what investigations do you wish to perform?*
- *On the assumption that the most likely diagnosis is idiopathic preterm labour, what initial management will you arrange? Give reasons for your actions.*
- *Three hours later her pain gets much worse and the cardiotocography is pathological. She was found on examination to be fully dilated with the head occipito-anterior 2 cm below the ischial spines. What would your subsequent management be?*

Notes on Your Approach to the Task

Examiner's Notes

Clearly this task centres on the diagnosis and management of idiopathic preterm labour. The competent candidate will initially wish to confirm the diagnosis by assessing whether the uterus is contracting and by performing a vaginal examination. If they are not specific about this, or need to be prompted by the examiner, it will be taken into account in the examiner's assessment of the candidate.

The examiner's questions have been written to allow the competent candidate to show how they reached a comprehensive differential diagnosis of either idiopathic preterm labour, urinary tract infection or abruption, and that they can apply their clinical knowledge to justify any relevant investigations such as an MSSU to rule out infection, or a CTG and ultrasound to look for signs of abruption.

Having reached the correct diagnosis, they will further demonstrate their applied clinical knowledge by giving a clear, evidence-based management plan, including steroids for lung maturation, and tocolytics to try to arrest the labour (even if only for long enough to allow the steroids to work). It is important to note in the third examiner's question, the word 'initial'. This should suggest to the competent candidate that a discussion of the management of the remaining eight weeks of the pregnancy is neither required nor expected.

The competent candidate's approach to the delivery of this patient is where this task would best test patient safety. The competent candidate would immediately realise that they need to discontinue the tocolysis, prepare the woman for immediate delivery by means of forceps, not ventouse, and so ensure there is good analgesia in the form of a pudendal block and perineal infiltration. The competent candidate will be able to describe to the examiner why it is inappropriate to delay delivery by undertaking a fetal blood sample, or to deliver by ventouse or by caesarean section.

In a case such as this, good communication with colleagues will take two broad forms. The first will be assessed by the examiner in the way the candidate interacts with him or her. The competent candidate will demonstrate clarity of thought and present their answers in a logical fashion without deviation from the point. They will be concise and precise in their approach, and show decisive decision-making when faced with what should be a relatively common scenario.

The second way communication skills will be assessed will be through the communication candidates recommend with other colleagues. Thus a competent candidate will warn the neonatal unit when this lady is first admitted, and ask the paediatricians to discuss the possible outlook should they be unable to stop the labour. Once the decision to deliver has been made, the competent candidate will ensure the paediatricians are in attendance, and the anaesthetic team forewarned in case of any difficulties such as major bleeding from an abruption.

Reflection on the Task

Review the notes you made before reading the examiner's notes. This is a communication task with a colleague, so it is acceptable to use medical terminology just as if you were discussing this case with your consultant on the labour ward.

- 'Justify' is a key word – you need to explain why you want to do a vaginal examination; just stating that you would do a VE won't achieve a pass.
- The emphasis is on clinical examination, so there is no credit for mentioning fetal fibronectin.
- You must mention stopping tocolysis or the examiner will assume you haven't done it.
- This task assesses working with the wider team as you must involve the neonatologists.

Module 8: Postpartum Problems (The Puerperium)

The puerperium is a stage of pregnancy in which obstetricians are rarely involved but is crucially important to mother and baby. Delivery of the baby is not the end of potential problems for either, and debriefing a mother after a difficult birth, once she has begun her recovery, can not only enhance her experience, but also prevent future misinterpretation of the facts, as well as complaints and litigation. Not only is it important to ensure the parents understand what happened, but the way issues are handled at such a time can have a huge impact for recovery and future pregnancies.

A review of module 12 of the core curriculum will clearly demonstrate that you must be able to both manage an uncomplicated mother and baby in the puerperium, including infant feeding, perineal tears and contraception, and also be able to manage abnormalities ranging from retained placenta to acute maternal collapse. From this latter perspective you would be expected to manage the delivery suite with distant support at night in many cases, and so must be able to provide all forms of emergency resuscitation until help arrives.

This module provides the opportunity to examine all five domains from acute obstetric management to debriefing and explanation to a patient with both clinical and lay examiners. An example task is given below.

Candidate's Instructions

This is a simulated patient task covering:

- *information gathering*
- *communication with patients*
- *patient safety*
- *applied clinical knowledge.*

You are an ST5 carrying out a morning ward round on the maternity ward. The midwife in charge is unhappy with the discharge note prepared by an FY2 for a patient who is about to go home. She has asked you to review the patient and ensure that the discharge arrangements are appropriate.

The case notes are not immediately available.

Women's Health Department
Queen Victoria Hospital
Manchester
MM1 0YM

DISCHARGE NOTE

Dear Dr Harrison,

Re: Helen Mills DOB: 19.4.1982

This 34-year-old woman was readmitted after her recent delivery and underwent a laparotomy. There was no internal bleeding, and group A streptococcus was grown from bacterial cultures. She was in intensive care for two days, and is now much better.

Yours sincerely

Dr Douglas

Foundation Doctor

You have ten minutes in which you should:

- *clarify the patient's recollection of events and concerns while awaiting the case notes*
- *explain group A streptococcus infection*
- *respond to her concerns*
- *explain what you will do to ensure safe transfer of care to the community*

Simulated Patient's Instructions

You are Helen Mills, a 34-year-old mother of three children, including your new baby, Annie. You have a four-year-old daughter who has just started school and a two-year-old son. Your daughter was a straightforward normal delivery and your son a planned caesarean section for a breech. You never had any other problems with your pregnancies. You were slightly worried about giving birth after a caesarean, but Annie was an easy delivery, and you went home after a day in hospital, partly because you were worried about your son, who was poorly with a cough and cold.

After a day at home you became very unwell and went back into hospital. You remember they were very worried about your blood pressure being so low and thought you were bleeding internally, so you were asked to sign a consent form for an operation. The next thing you remember was coming round in intensive care. You were told that they found pus in your belly and you now have a large wound up and down your tummy.

This was a frightening experience with buzzers and alarms going off the whole time. Though the staff were kind and tried to explain what was going on, you found it impossible to take things in. You breastfed your other children but were too ill for that to be possible this time and are disappointed about that too.

Two days ago you were transferred back to the maternity ward, where the midwives seemed so busy looking after the other mothers with new babies that you still aren't sure what has happened to you, and now they have said you are to go home.

You are a slightly nervous person, and you are aware that you were near death on intensive care and have lost confidence in your ability to cope.

If not covered by the candidate, you could ask the following questions:

- *What is this germ that nearly killed me?*
- *Where did I catch this germ? The toilets didn't look very clean and I really think that it's your dirty hospital that made me so ill.*
- *How do I know that I will be safe at home?*
- *What will happen next?*

Acting requirements:

- *You will be very nervous, but keen to get home to your baby.*
- *You will be fearful of returning to hospital.*
- *You will not yet be thinking of the next pregnancy.*

Notes on Your Approach to the Task

Examiner's Notes

As can be seen, very little information has been provided, so the competent candidate will begin to consider what questions they will need to ask to get the required information while awaiting the buzzer to call them in.

The competent candidate will quickly establish what the woman remembers, and using their knowledge of septicaemic shock will soon begin to deliver a likely and plausible explanation of what happened using terms the woman can understand. The competent candidate will not be able to say for certain that their description is correct, but may use terms like 'it is most likely that . . .' or 'the most probable explanation is . . .', offering to check once the records become available. With the information the actor has been asked to provide and what is written in the letter, it should not be difficult to reach a likely chronology of events and explanation.

A scenario such as this offers the candidate ample opportunity to demonstrate their communication skills with patients. First, the woman will need to be put at ease if she is to impart the information the candidate needs. She will need an explanation of what happened in clear and plain English, avoiding clinical or technical terms. In addition, a good candidate will say they are sorry this has happened but that it probably could not have been avoided. There will be an overlap with patient safety to ensure she is given sufficient information regarding what to look out for over the coming days and weeks, without frightening her. It is important to ensure she does not blame herself or her son, who most likely was the original source of the infection. She will also need to be reassured without hiding the truth from her. While many common conditions will have pre-prepared information leaflets, it's unlikely that a unit will have one to cover an unusual scenario such as this, so it is doubtful that a candidate will receive any credit from the examiners for 'offering leaflets'.

As far as patient safety is concerned, now the acute episode is over the important issue will be to ensure she continues any medication she may have been prescribed (particularly antibiotics, which a competent candidate will probably check as soon as the records become available, rather than assuming they have been prescribed). It will be important to give accurate advice on what to expect over the coming days and weeks in terms of not only the birth and newborn baby, but also both the laparotomy and the infection. In addition, the competent candidate will advise that she asks her GP to check the children in case they have an infection that needs treating. The competent candidate will not press her on future pregnancies at this stage, but will arrange a further appointment as an out-patient to discuss this, at which she can bring her partner and may well be more receptive to such information. The woman can be reassured that there will be an internal investigation to see if anything could have been done to prevent this, and whether there are any lessons for other mothers for the future.

A competent candidate will apply their clinical knowledge to build up a picture of the likely scenario and course of events to understand what has happened to this lady. They will then use that knowledge to demonstrate that they can safely and effectively manage the patient, and send her home to her family in the confident knowledge that she is over the worst of her problems, but should anything further happen she has the ability to contact her midwife or the delivery unit to ask for further help and reassurance.

As can be seen, this scenario offers many opportunities to assess the ST5 in all five domains. If the notes were provided, the candidate could have a similar discussion with the consultant over what has happened to test communication with colleagues. They could also be required to write an appropriate discharge letter assessing written communication.

Reflection on the Task

Review the notes you made before reading the examiner's notes. Did you understand that the purpose of this task is to assess information gathering and provide an explanation while acknowledging you cannot be certain until you see the notes?

- Communication with primary care is essential after serious clinical problems such as septicaemia.
- The GP may need to treat the wider family for Strep. A.
- You need to reassure the patient while ensuring she understands exactly what happened to her.

Module 9: Gynaecological Problems

General benign gynaecology symptoms, including menstrual disorders, pelvic pain and vaginal discharge, are common presenting symptoms to any gynaecologist, and as such you should be able to manage them easily and efficiently. In addition, this module includes the management of emergency gynaecology, most of which you should be able to manage independently by the time you have reached ST5 and are attempting your Part 3 exam.

When you read this module of the curriculum, you will also see some less common conditions are included, such as congenital abnormalities of the genital tract, paediatric gynaecology and puberty. More common conditions include endocrine disorders as they apply to gynaecology and the menopause.

If this varied list of pathology is combined with all five domains, you can see that you could be examined on a condition you may see every day at work, or on something you have never seen, for which you will need to rely on theoretical knowledge. Equally, the task could be set as a straightforward approach such as managing a simulated patient with menopausal symptoms, or in an unexpected manner such as counselling a patient who requests HRT for a premature ovarian failure but has breast cancer. The important thing to realise is that you will be assessed not just on how you approach the task, but against the standard expected by the examiners of a trainee at ST5 level. In other words, the examiner's expectations for your management plan would be greater if the task was based on a common condition, and lower if it was a rare one. In the latter case the examiner would be expecting a more reassuring approach, with good communication and assurance to the patient that, having sought further advice, you will ensure it is communicated to them. You will have to decide the best approach in the two minutes you have to read the candidate's information.

An example of a question that covers a small aspect of this module is given below.

Candidate's Instructions

This is a simulated patient task assessing:

- *information gathering*
- *communication with patients*
- *patient safety*
- *applied clinical knowledge.*

You are an ST5 working in the gynaecology clinic. You are about to see the patient whose referral letter from her general practitioner is as follows.

> *Gaywood Road Surgery*
> *Norwich*
> *NR7 4SE*

Dear Doctor,

Re: Karen Dent

Could you please arrange to see this 17-year-old girl who has been troubled with pelvic pain over the last eight months?
The pain is interfering with her normal daily activities as well as school attendance. She has used different pain killers with no benefit. She is concerned about the persistence of pain and would like to discuss this matter with you.

Yours sincerely,

Mohamed Faris

Dr M Faris MRCGP

You have ten minutes in which you should:

- *take a relevant history*
- *explain the most likely causes of her pelvic pain*
- *discuss possible investigations to reach a diagnosis*
- *answer Karen's questions and address her concerns*

Simulated Patient's Instructions

You are Karen Dent, aged 17 years. You are still studying at school and hope to go to university next year. You have pain in your lower tummy, and are concerned that it will interfere with your ability to pass your upcoming exams. You live with your parents.

You started having periods at the age of 13 and your periods, although regular, have always been painful. You have a boyfriend but you are not sexually active with him. You should become 'shy but honest' when asked about any sexual activity with your boyfriend because at the age of seven you were sexually abused by a close relative but you prefer not to talk about it. Do not be too forthcoming about this but mention it if the candidate asks about it in a direct but sympathetic way.

You have always had lower abdominal pain, but it has got worse over the last eight months. The pain is usually dull but can be sharp on occasions. The pain doesn't follow any particular pattern and you are not aware of anything that can make it better or worse. If asked, it is not related to your periods. You have no urinary or bowel symptoms. You don't sleep well because of the pain and you are under a lot of pressure from your parents and teachers because of the impact of the pain on your school work and attendance.

You have tried several pain killers, both over the counter and prescribed by your GP, but they didn't touch the pain. You started to take the combined oral contraceptive 'Loestrin® 20' last cycle but are not keen on continuing as there was no significant benefit. You have never had an operation.

Your mother suffers from endometriosis and had several treatments before having a hysterectomy at the age of 38. Your older sister also suffers from endometriosis and had fertility treatment to conceive.

You wish to know the cause of your pain and in particular if you have endometriosis.

If not covered by the candidate, you could ask the following questions:

- *What are the possible causes of my pain?*
- *Could it be 'endometriosis' like my mother and sister?*

Notes on Your Approach to the Task

Examiner's Notes

It can immediately be seen that this is a relatively common presentation that an ST5 would be expected to have encountered very frequently, so the expectation of the examiners will be that the competent candidate will be able to manage the consultation largely independently. The key point here is that while the obvious differential diagnosis is endometriosis, the symptoms do not fit a typical pattern, which should alert the competent candidate to look for other causes.

The competent candidate will take a brief and targeted history, and soon identify that the pain is far more longstanding than the GP has said, that it is unrelated to her cycle and not relieved by analgesics. They will ask specific questions to rule out other organic causes of her pain. They should then pick up on her change of attitude when asking about whether she is sexually active with her boyfriend, which will then allow them to enquire sympathetically about any possible abuse.

The manner in which the competent candidate communicates with the patient will be crucial as to whether they develop a rapport with her, and hence whether she informs them of the history of abuse. The candidate who is too 'matter of fact' will build barriers. She is a vulnerable girl with what is to her a distressing secret, so the competent candidate will make use of the clues she gives them, apologise for having to ask difficult questions, then ask in such a way that she can begin to admit the abuse.

Applied clinical knowledge will be assessed by the way the competent candidate approaches the differential diagnosis. They will explain why the symptoms lack the characteristics of endometriosis (e.g. pelvic pain of cyclic pattern), but agree that this does not exclude the diagnosis. They will acknowledge that there is an increased risk of endometriosis because of her family history. A brief review of other possible causes of pelvic pain, including bowel or urinary causes which are also less likely, will lead to the possibility of either a psychological cause following the abuse, or perhaps adhesions secondary to infection at the time of the abuse.

Under the domain of patient safety, the competent candidate will explain that the contraceptive pill is not likely to help her pain, but is important should she be considering becoming sexually active. The competent candidate will realise that they are unqualified to provide the counselling required to help such a patient (this would not be expected of an ST5), and will therefore suggest referral to a counsellor. In addition, having identified the history of abuse, the competent candidate will be aware of their obligations to this vulnerable patient under Safeguarding.

This patient wants an answer to the cause of her pain, yet the competent candidate will not rush to perform a diagnostic laparoscopy as there is significant chance it will be normal. Therefore, there should be an element of negotiation, perhaps offering to take swabs for infection and checking a pelvic ultrasound to delay the need for a laparoscopy until after she has seen a counsellor, if her pain is not settling. These are difficult conversations, but the competent candidate's ability to bring these issues into the open will again be a measure of their skills in communicating with patients.

Reflection on the Task

Review the notes that you made before reading the examiner's notes. Did you think about exam technique to realise that chronic pelvic pain is such a common condition that there must be a hidden agenda for it to feature as a task in the Part 3 exam?

- History-taking needs to cover non-gynaecological causes too.
- Practise a statement that 'gives the patient permission' to disclose abuse.
- Use your communication skills to convey sensitivity without embarrassment.
- Remember that the Green-top Guideline advises against laparoscopy as the first-line for investigating chronic pelvic pain.

Module 10: Subfertility

A clear understanding of the investigation, diagnosis and management of the common causes of subfertility, along with the legal and ethical issues they raise, are essential for any gynaecologist.

A review of the core curriculum module will reveal that, to be able to understand the investigation of subfertility, you will need to be able to order the correct endocrine investigations at the correct time, be able to interpret routine imaging and be competent to perform both diagnostic hysteroscopy and diagnostic laparoscopy. As part of a diagnostic laparoscopy this module also requires you to be able to assess and stage endometriosis. Your practical ability to undertake these procedures is likely to have been assessed through the relevant workplace-based assessments, but some of those skills could still be examined in the Part 3 exam through a risk management or teaching task.

While an ability to perform the various procedures of assisted conception, such as ovulation induction, IVF, ICSI or gamete donation, could be expected to be learned in the senior training years after attaining the MRCOG, in order to pass the Part 3 exam you would be expected to have a working knowledge of the indications and procedures in order to allow you to counsel appropriately, within your limitations, patients who are being referred on to a fertility unit.

Alongside the physical issues of managing the infertile couple, in the setting of healthcare in the UK, there is specific advice about provision of services that you should be aware of, published by NICE and the Scottish Guidelines Network. In addition, it is important for the MRCOG examination as a whole, not just Part 3, that you understand and have an empathetic approach to the issues raised by same-sex partnerships and single parenthood.

The area frequently forgotten when looking at subfertility is the impact many chronic conditions may have on fertility. You should be aware that a history of conditions such as cancer, major abdominal surgery or eating disorders can impact on a woman's ability to conceive; you should be able to advise the patient appropriately when they present to your gynaecology clinic.

The psychological impact on some couples of not being able to have a child can be immense; you should always bear this in mind when managing them, and ensure you have a sympathetic but objective approach. A typical example of the sort of task you might encounter in the Part 3 exam is shown below.

Candidate's Instructions

This is a simulated patient task assessing:

- *communication with patients*
- *information gathering*
- *applied clinical knowledge*
- *patient safety.*

You are an ST5 in gynaecology out-patients and are about to see Mrs Mary McNoughton, who has been referred with a fertility problem. The referral letter is provided for you to read:

> *The GP Surgery*
> *High Street*
> *Marylebone*
> *London*

Dear Gynaecologist

Re: Mary McNoughton – 40 Regent's Park, London.

> *I would be most grateful if you could please see this 37-year-old woman who is requesting donor insemination fertility treatment as a single parent. She has a tragic history. Her husband was killed in a road traffic accident while she was pregnant and she now lives with her two-year-old son. She makes the point that she would not wish her son to grow up as an only child and that her chances of meeting a new partner in her situation are remote.*
> *She is otherwise fit and well. I have checked her progesterone levels and your laboratory have reported them as ovulatory.*
> *Thank you for your help.*

Yours sincerely

A. Mohammed

Dr Ahmed Mohammed FRCGP

You have ten minutes in which you should:

- *obtain the relevant facts regarding the patient's request*
- *deal with the patient's concerns and answer her questions*

Simulated Patient's Instructions

You are Mary McNoughton, aged 37 years. You are requesting fertility treatment as a single parent. You married when you were 30 and always wanted at least two children. You conceived within six months of trying with your first pregnancy, but then tragically your husband was killed in a road traffic accident while you were still pregnant, so he never saw his son. You went on to have a normal vaginal delivery and now live with your two-year-old son, Luke. You have no financial problems.

You remain very sad about the loss of your husband but realise that life must go on. In particular, you do not want Luke to be an only child. You and your husband were both from large families; you remain close to both families and meet regularly. You also have a close circle of friends, including male friends, but realise that your chance of finding a new partner to share life with Luke and yourself is remote and this is not what you want to do. Family and friends are supportive of your desire for another child.

Your general practitioner has suggested donor insemination as a means of conceiving.

You are otherwise fit and well. Your periods started when you were 12 and your cycle has always been reasonably regular, varying from 28 to about 31 days. The only time you have been in hospital was to have your baby.

If not covered by the candidate, you could ask the following questions:

- *What are my chances of being accepted for treatment?*
- *What are my chances of having a child?*
- *Who will be the legal father?*
- *What tests will I need?*
- *Is there a problem finding donors?*
- *Do I have any alternatives?*

Notes on Your Approach to the Task

Examiner's Notes

This task is designed to test the candidate's knowledge of fertility treatment and their ability to communicate this to a patient who is making a request with profound ethical and legal implications. They should conduct the interview in a non-judgemental and supportive manner, but remain realistic in their advice.

Within information gathering, the competent candidate will obviously need to ensure they obtain the relevant additional facts from the patient, particularly around her previous conception. Credit will not be given for confirming the information given in the GP letter, although this is provided as a signpost to the competent candidate of the issues they are likely to need to address. It is also important that the competent candidate enquires about her social support – as she will need help once the baby is born – as well as her financial security as it is unlikely donor insemination will be funded by the NHS. All of these factors are also important in assessing how well this woman has thought through her request.

This lady will be vulnerable, and an ability to communicate sympathetically yet knowledgeably with her will be vital. The competent candidate will not use technical terms, nor will they promise that her request will be successful. The competent candidate will make her aware that even if she is accepted by a fertility unit, there has been a shortage of donors in the UK since the donor's right to anonymity was removed. The competent candidate will also need to inform the woman that if a donor is found, there is only a 10 per cent chance of conception, and if she is successful she will have to put 'unknown' on the baby's birth certificate as the father.

In applying clinical knowledge, the competent candidate will demonstrate their understanding that although donor insemination is legal in the UK, there may still be ethical issues to be dealt with as the welfare of the potential child is paramount. It is likely she will need to see a counsellor before treatment is given.

Within the patient safety domain, the competent candidate will be aware that she will need to be checked for routine communicable diseases such as HIV, hepatitis B and C and rubella. In addition, she will need to have her tubal patency checked, but this can be done using a hysterosalpingogram rather than by laparoscopy, in order to avoid an anaesthetic. In addition, the competent candidate will reassure her regarding the steps taken by the infertility unit to reduce the risks of contracting any infectious disease, including HIV, from the donor.

There is a lot to get through in this task, and while the competent candidate may not be able to cover it all, they may still achieve the standard required. A good candidate may also discuss other options available to her, such as finding a new partner or seeking a donor from among her acquaintances. Adoption or even reproductive tourism will have significant implications for both communication and patient safety, but it would not be essential to cover all of these areas to pass this task.

Reflection on the Task

Review the notes you made before reading the examiner's notes. Did you understand that this task assesses more than just clinical knowledge and how to investigate and treat with donor sperm?

- Ethical issues are key, as the welfare of the potential child must be considered in all assisted conception.
- Do you understand the legal issues about screening of donors?
- Practise a non-judgemental approach to single parenthood.
- You must gently challenge the patient to consider other options.

Module 11: Sexual and Reproductive Health

A clear understanding of contraception, termination of pregnancy and sexual health are fundamental to a career in obstetrics and gynaecology. If you review the contents of this module you will realise that it is essential to understand the principles of contraception and you will be expected to be able to counsel a woman and her partner about the various options available to them. In order to do this you will need to be able to have potentially sensitive conversations with them about their sexual needs and all aspects of family planning. On the other hand, the sexual health needs of vulnerable women such as young people, sex workers and drug users will be different and therefore require a different approach.

You will also note this module includes termination of pregnancy. It is important that you understand your obligations under UK law irrespective of your personal views. The issue of termination of pregnancy may well arise in this module or even module 4 (antenatal care), and it is important that you deal with any such clinical situation in a sympathetic but objective manner.

This is one clinical area that will often require a multidisciplinary approach. You need to be aware of the other care workers who could be involved in a woman's care, and understand when they should be involved with her permission, and potentially when they should be involved without her permission if you are dealing with a Safeguarding issue.

Below is an example of a task covering this module.

Candidate's Instructions

This task is a structured discussion covering:

- *information gathering*
- *applied clinical knowledge*
- *patient safety.*

You are the ST5 on call and you were asked to assess Mrs Melanie White, a 42-year-old woman who presented to the Emergency Department with suprapubic pain and feeling unwell.

The pain started one week ago and has got progressively worse. She tried simple pain killers that helped initially but not anymore. She saw her GP two days ago, and he prescribed codeine to no effect. Today the pain has become very severe and she fainted, developed diarrhoea and vomiting and felt feverish.

Mrs White lives with her husband and three children, aged 14, 10 and 7 years, all born vaginally. She had an IUCD inserted three years ago and has regular but heavy periods. Her last menstrual period was three weeks ago. She has no other medical history of note.

The examiner will have a conversation with you based on a series of questions, and will provide you with further relevant information as the discussion progresses. The examiner will guide you on timings.

You have ten minutes in which you should:

- *read the information provided*
- *answer the questions asked by the examiner*

Examiner's Instructions

Familiarise yourself with the candidate's instructions.

Use the following three questions as a basis for a discussion with the candidate about the management of this patient. As you approach the last question, show the candidate the observation chart.

- *What initial information and initial investigations would you like to base your management on?*
- *Examination reveals a large abdomino-pelvic mass, a very tender abdomen with guarding and rigidity, no cervical excitation and no offensive discharge. Her pregnancy test is negative. Describe your immediate management of Mrs White.*
- *You have now given intravenous fluids, oxygen and antibiotics. Her white cell count and C-reactive protein are raised. An ultrasound scan shows a large left-sided pelvic mass of mixed echogenicity measuring 12 × 10 × 9 cm separate from a normal uterus containing an IUCD. A small volume of free fluid is seen in the pelvis. Based on the updated observation chart and results of investigations, what would you do next?*

NEWS KEY 0 1 2 3	NAME: Melanie White	D.O.B. 24/3/74	ADMISSION DATE: 20/5/16

	DATE	20/5	20/5	20/5								DATE
	TIME	15:15	9:30	8:45	10:00	10:15						TIME

RESP. RATE
≥25		•	•			3			≥25
21-24	•	•	•			2			21-24
12-20									12-20
9-11						1			9-11
≤8						3			≤8

SpO₂
≥96	•								≥96
94-95		•	•			1			94-95
92-93			•			2			92-93
≤91				•		3			≤91
Inspired O₂ %						2			%

TEMP
≥39°	•	•				2			≥39°
38°						1			38°
37°		•							37°
36°			•						36°
≤35°				•		1			≤35°
						3			

BLOOD PRESSURE (NEW SCORE uses Systolic BP)
230						3			230
220									220
210									210
200									200
190									190
180									180
170									170
160									160
150									150
140									140
130									130
120									120
110	∧ ∧					1			110
100		∧ ∧ ∧				2			100
90									90
80									80
70						3			70
60									60
50									50

HEART RATE
>140						3			140
130			•	•		2			130
120		•	•						120
110		•				1			110
100	•								100
90									90
80									80
70									70
60									60
50						1			50
40									40
30						3			30

Level of Consciousness	Alert	•	•	•						Alert
	V / P / U			•	•	3				V / P / U

BLOOD SUGAR									Bl'd Sugar

TOTAL NEW SCORE	5	7	7	12	15				TOTAL SCORE

Additional Parameters
Pain Score									Pain Score
Urine Output									Urine Output
Monitoring Frequency									Monitor Freq
Escalation Plan Y/N n/a									Escal Plan
Initials									Initials

National Early Warning Score: July 2012

Figure 3.3

┌───┐
│   │
│ Notes on Your Approach to the Task   │
│   │
│   │
│   │
│   │
│   │
│   │
│   │
│   │
│   │
│   │
│   │
│   │
│   │
│   │
└───┘

Examiner's Notes

This scenario assesses the candidate's ability to diagnose and manage an acute pelvic abscess. The competent candidate will realise that the history has already been given to them so the information they will need to gather will relate to her observations, such as her level of consciousness, heart rate, blood pressure, temperature, respiratory rate, oxygen saturation, abdominal tenderness, presence of any pelvic masses and results of her pelvic examination in order to help them reach a diagnosis.

The competent candidate will then apply their clinical knowledge to ask for a number of investigations, such as a full blood count and C-reactive protein, arterial blood gases, and renal and liver function tests. As this woman could be very unwell they should check for evidence of infection by means of appropriate swabs, looking for both sexually transmitted organisms and organisms that may be related to her IUCD. In addition, blood cultures would be justifiable. The competent candidate would also ask the woman to provide a specimen of urine, in order not only to check for infection, but also to ensure she is not pregnant. Finally, if there is any doubt about the examination findings, an urgent ultrasound would be sensible. A candidate who mentions tumour markers would not necessarily receive any credit, as although this woman could have ovarian pathology, the examiner will assess their response against the words 'initial' and 'immediate', which would therefore not be appropriate. However, a candidate who said they would send the sample while they were taking blood from the patient in case tumour markers were needed may get some credit.

This woman is extremely sick, and by describing a prompt, clear, appropriate management plan the competent candidate will ensure she is kept clinically safe. The competent candidate will initially resuscitate and manage her by administering intravenous fluids and broad spectrum antibiotics, preferably with the advice of a microbiologist. Mrs White will need anti-pyretics and oxygen initially, but if her condition continues to deteriorate the competent candidate will realise that if she is not responding to conservative treatment, she may need a laparotomy, which would be outside the competencies of an ST5 to undertake independently. They should therefore inform the consultant gynaecologist to prepare for a possible laparotomy and removal of her IUCD. It would also be important that the possible need for high-dependency care after the procedure is discussed with the anaesthetist pre-operatively.

Reflection on the Task

Review the notes you made before reading the examiner's notes. In this structured discussion the examiner will ask a series of questions and it is essential to listen carefully. The questions mention initial information, initial investigations and immediate management. This warns you that your answers need to be specific to the acute situation; you won't gain any credit for developing a long-term plan.

- Practise how you would explain the need to screen for STIs to a patient in a long-term relationship if this were a simulated patient task.
- Consider patient safety in the management of acute sepsis.

Module 12: Early Pregnancy Care

The care of women in uncomplicated early pregnancy is covered in module 4, antenatal care. This module looks at all aspects of the care of women with abnormalities of early pregnancy, from threatened miscarriage through ectopic pregnancy to trophoblastic disease. As can be seen, this represents a wide range of clinical scenarios on which you could be examined across all five domains.

As early pregnancy is a very emotional time for a pregnant woman and her partner, you are very likely to be assessed in your communication skills, in particular in the way you break bad news and counsel a woman about what may be some very difficult options and decisions that you are asking her to make.

As an ST5 you would be expected to manage most complications of early pregnancy independently, so the standard expected of you by the examiners will reflect this. In addition, you may need to offer advice about the investigation and treatment of other medical conditions in the first trimester, in particular those with which you are not familiar. Even so, your advice should be sensible and objective, and you should ensure you signpost the woman and her partner to a more appropriate clinician if necessary.

An example of the type of task you may encounter in the module is shown below.

Candidate's Instructions

This task is a structured discussion covering:

- *information gathering*
- *applied clinical knowledge*
- *patient safety*
- *communication with patients.*

You are the ST5 on call and have been told that a 31-year-old has been admitted to the Emergency Department with a 24-hour history of minor painless vaginal bleeding in her first pregnancy. She also says she has been vomiting almost constantly for the past five days. Her last menstrual period was ten weeks ago and she has had a positive pregnancy test. You have been asked to see her for a gynaecology opinion. The results of an initial blood profile performed by the emergency doctors are shown in Table 3.2.

Table 3.2

Haematocrit	36%	(35–47%)
Haemoglobin	117 g/l	(110–160 g/l)
Sodium	127 mmol/l	(133–145 mmol/l)
Potassium	3.0 mmol/l	(3.5–5.3 mmol/l)
Chloride	93 mmol/l	(95–108 mmol/l)
Albumin	36 g/dl	(37–49 g/dl)
Urea	7.9 mmol/l	(2.5–7.8 mmol/l)
Bilirubin	18 µmol/l	(0–20 µmol/l)
GGT	37 µmol/l	(4–35 µmol/l)
ALT	57 µmol/l	(8–55 µmol/l)
Alk Phos	110 µmol/l	(30–130 µmol/l)
Blood group	A Rhesus negative	

The examiner will have a conversation with you based on a series of questions, and will provide you with further relevant information as the discussion progresses. The examiner will guide you on timings.

You have ten minutes in which you should:

- *read the information provided*
- *answer the questions asked by the examiner*

Examiner's Instructions

Familiarise yourself with the candidate's instructions.

Use the following five questions as a basis for a discussion with the candidate about the management of this patient. After the candidate has addressed the third question below, give the candidate the scan result.

- *What additional clinical information would you require and what would be your initial management?*
- *If asked by the candidate, say the uterus is of 16-week size with no adnexal tenderness and urinalysis shows ketonuria ++++.*
- *What further investigations would you undertake once the patient is admitted?*
- *How will you manage the patient in the short term and why?*
- *How should this patient be managed after the pregnancy, and what should she be told?*

Ultrasound Scan

Transvaginal scan of pelvis undertaken – good views obtained.
Uterus enlarged for gestation, but no identifiable fetus seen.
Only vesicular tissue is identified and appears as a snowstorm, suggestive of a complete hydatidiform mole.
Ovaries are partially cystic, but within the normal range in dimension.

Notes on Your Approach to the Task

Examiner's Notes

Even a competent candidate is likely to initially treat this woman as having a threatened miscarriage, with an element of hyperemesis gravidarum. In order to reach that diagnosis, however, the competent candidate will need to seek additional information from the patient and the Emergency Department team, such as the severity of her vomiting and whether she has any other gastrointestinal symptoms to suggest something such as gastroenteritis. It addition, they would seek clarity of whether this might be due to a urinary tract infection or whether she has taken any medication. Once the competent candidate is aware of the examination findings and has ascertained that there is ketonuria, this should confirm a diagnosis of hyperemesis gravidarum.

Having reached the diagnosis, the competent candidate will initially apply their clinical knowledge to manage the hyperemesis by means of rehydration with intravenous fluids and antiemetics to try to control the sickness. They will describe an acceptable regimen as this should be everyday practice for them. Thereafter, they should plan to monitor the hyperemesis by means of daily urinalysis; if it does not respond to first-line treatment they should move on to second-line, such as a 5HT3 receptor antagonist (ondansetron) or steroids.

When assessing the competent candidate's approach to patient safety, the first thing they should organise once the patient is admitted is an ultrasound scan to rule out multiple or molar pregnancy. At that point the examiner will share the ultrasound report, which will confirm the diagnosis. This is the moment when the competent candidate can first justify requesting a serum hCG, as there was no indication for it prior to this in the chronology. They will then need to explain the findings to the patient first, and should recommend suction curettage rather than medical treatment due to the risk of dissemination of trophoblastic tissue. In addition, the competent candidate will explain that cervical preparation should not be used for the same reason.

In order to address the last of the examiner's comments, the competent candidate will revert to demonstration of their applied clinical knowledge. They should be aware that there is no requirement for anti-D as there are no fetal blood cells. They should also be aware of the management protocols for trophoblastic disease in the UK, so the patient should be registered with an identified screening centre for follow-up of hCG levels (blood/urine) for a minimum of six months.

Finally, the competent candidate will be able to clearly describe the advice that should be communicated to the patient, in particular to avoid pregnancy using a barrier method of contraception for at least six months and until hCG levels have returned to normal. The competent candidate will signpost the patient to written information about trophoblastic disease such as the RCOG leaflet, and should emphasise that any subsequent pregnancy should be evaluated at an early stage by ultrasound and the hCG levels checked by the screening centre 6–8 weeks after the end of the pregnancy to exclude disease recurrence.

Reflection on the Task

Review the notes you made before reading the examiner's notes. Did you think about the principles of exam technique? Hyperemesis is such a common condition that it should have been obvious that there would be something unusual about this case and you should have spotted that it's likely the scenario would be about multiple pregnancy or molar pregnancy.

- Ensure you understand the reporting and monitoring arrangements for molar pregnancy in the UK.
- Be specific when asking for additional information.
- Make sure you give information about molar pregnancy, such as not needing anti-D; it's easy to forget the important negatives.

Module 13: Gynaecological Oncology

Generally speaking, most operative gynaecological oncology is learned following attainment of the MRCOG during either subspecialist training or if undertaking an advanced training skills module (ATSM). However as an ST5 you will be expected to not only understand the anatomy and pathology of gynaecological cancer, but also be able to tell patients the results of their investigations and what they can expect as they enter one of the cancer pathways. A clear knowledge of the cancer targets in the UK is therefore essential.

In order to meet the standards of this module, you will need to understand pre-malignant disease and its implications, the classification of various gynaecological cancers and the principles of treatment. In particular, you will need to be able to recognise and plan the management of premalignant disease of the vulva, cervix and endometrium, and malignant disease of the vulva, cervix, endometrium and ovary. Your ability to counsel patients in such situations with care and sympathy – yet not concealing the truth – will be very easy to assess through a consultation with a simulated patient within this module.

Do not underestimate the psychological component of this module. You will need to be able to break bad news to very vulnerable patients and their families at a time when many will hear the word cancer and immediately panic. You will also need to be able to explain difficult treatments, many of which will have positive benefits; however, you may also be asked to discuss treatment failures and even impending death.

In addition, a key component of this module is the role of the multidisciplinary team (MDT). This term was first coined in cancer services as a means of ensuring adherence to the latest treatment guidelines and the highest possible standards of care. In cancer the MDT is not just about the different medical specialties, but also includes cancer nurse specialists in particular, and so in approaching this module you will need to understand each individual's role and how they combine to enhance both outcomes and experience for the patient.

As can be seen from the Part 3 clinical assessment template (Appendix 1), this module also includes many aspects of surgical safety and clinical governance that are also included in other modules.

An example task is given below.

Candidate's Instructions

This is a simulated patient task assessing:

- *communication with patients*
- *information gathering*
- *applied clinical knowledge*
- *patient safety.*

You are an ST5 and you are about to see a 46-year-old woman who had a vaginal hysterectomy three weeks ago. The patient has been brought back to clinic unexpectedly because of the histopathology report, which is shown below.

Histopathology Report

Mrs Jane Perton
Hospital No.: X007077072
SPECIMEN UTERUS AND CERVIX
The endometrium shows areas of atypical hyperplasia but also shows foci of a well-differentiated endometrioid adenocarcinoma of grade 1. Foci of squamous metaplasia are present and in some areas the glandular structures contain aggregations of neutrophils. Nuclear enlargement and pleomorphism are generally mild. The lesion is generally well-defined and shows only minimal invasion into the myometrium, less than 1 mm. Separation by at least 11 mm from the superior serosal surface is confirmed. No lympho-vascular permeation is seen. The presence of a benign leiomyoma is confirmed. The cervix is free from tumour and is unremarkable.

You have ten minutes in which you should:

- *obtain a brief targeted history*
- *explain the histopathology result*
- *establish and answer the patient's concerns*
- *outline and justify a management plan*

Simulated Patient's Instructions

You are Mrs Jane Perton, a 46-year-old nurse. You have been in a stable relationship with John, a 50-year-old businessman, for 20 years. You are both in good health, do not smoke, only occasionally drink alcohol and lead healthy lifestyles. You do not have any allergies. You have always had regular smears and they have always been normal. You have had two normal deliveries in the past.

You had a vaginal hysterectomy three weeks ago because of heavy and regular periods. You have never had any bleeding after sex, but had some spotting a couple of months ago in between your periods, which you assumed you could safely ignore. Your ovaries were not removed.

Prior to the operation you had tried various tablets both during your period and in the run up to it, none of which had helped. You were offered alternative treatments but chose to proceed with a hysterectomy as you had become aware of a lump protruding through the vagina over the last few months, which the doctor had said was an early prolapse.

A biopsy of the lining of your womb carried out four months before the operation was reported as normal. When you were discharged from hospital you were told that the operation had gone well and that there was no need for you to come back to hospital for follow-up. You have not had any problems since the operation.

You are attending the gynaecology clinic today because you have recently received a letter enclosing an appointment. You have attended on your own and do not know why you have been asked to attend, but should act as though you are very worried.

If not covered by the candidate, you could ask the following questions:

- *Why have I been asked to come back to the clinic?*
- *Do I need any more treatment?*
- *Do I need to see anyone else?*
- *Do I have cancer?*
- *Has the cancer spread?*
- *Why didn't the biopsy identify the cancer?*
- *What happens next?*

```
┌─────────────────────────────────────────────────────────────────────────┐
│  Notes on Your Approach to the Task                                        │
│                                                                           │
│                                                                           │
│                                                                           │
│                                                                           │
│                                                                           │
│                                                                           │
│                                                                           │
│                                                                           │
│                                                                           │
│                                                                           │
│                                                                           │
│                                                                           │
│                                                                           │
└─────────────────────────────────────────────────────────────────────────┘
```

Examiner's Notes

It is important that early in the consultation the competent candidate finds out what the patient already knows or suspects, so they can ensure the patient has all the information they need to be able to explain the diagnosis and initial steps in further investigation and treatment. In doing this they will ascertain that the hysterectomy was done for failed medical treatment of heavy and regular periods, that all her cervical smears have been normal, as was the endometrial biopsy four months before the hysterectomy. This will give the good candidate an opportunity to explain to the patient that even if all investigations have been normal it is still possible to have endometrial cancer as the previous biopsy may not have sampled the whole cavity and the cancer may be confined to a small area.

One of the key domains this task assesses is communication with patients. The first thing the competent candidate will need to do is explain in simple terms to the patient exactly what the histology has unexpectedly shown, namely cancer of the lining of the womb. While it is accepted practice, particularly at medical student level, to discuss potentially malignant diagnoses without using the term cancer, when breaking such news to a patient like this, it is important to be explicit as otherwise there is a risk they will leave the consultation thinking: 'I don't know what an endometrioid adenocarcinoma is, but what a relief the doctor did not say I had cancer.' That said, the competent candidate will need to come across as caring, empathetic and, while objective, will neither be unnecessarily optimistic nor pessimistic. They will make every endeavour to develop a rapport with the patient. Although there are only ten minutes for this task, the competent candidate should not talk constantly, but give the patient opportunities to gather her thoughts and ask questions.

The competent candidate will be able to interpret the histology result for the patient by applying their clinical knowledge of both the pathology and the possible treatment. They will be able to explain that the tumour appears to be at an early stage and at this time appears small and confined to the womb, which has already been removed. In addition there is only superficial invasion and no invasion of blood vessels or lymphatics, all of which can be seen as positive, although until further scans (MRI) have been completed the candidate cannot be certain, and should say so. If, however, this is confirmed, the outlook is good with five-year survival rates in the region of 90%.

From a patient safety perspective the competent candidate will explain the principles of the cancer MDT, and the need to discuss the histology and further imaging before making a definitive management plan. In addition, the competent candidate will explain that these tumours can be stimulated by oestrogen and so it will be important to remove her ovaries, but this can be done laparoscopically to make her recovery easier. If the MRI shows evidence of lymphadenopathy this can be addressed at the same time. In answer to her question about further treatment, the competent candidate should explain that this will depend on many factors, and that while she may need radiotherapy, for many patients the initial surgery is sufficient.

The competent candidate will realise the patient will not know the diagnosis, and so will explore whether they are alone, and whether they wish to return with their partner so they too can understand the implications of the diagnosis.

Reflection on the Task

Review the notes you made before reading the examiner's notes. In this task, time management will be key as there is a lot to be covered in ten minutes.

- Practise an opening statement to explain that you need to ask a few questions before discussing the histology result in order to signpost the consultation.
- The instruction to take a brief targeted history is a warning not to waste time.
- Give a warning shot that you are about to break bad news then objectively give the diagnosis.
- It is okay to use the word cancer; don't use euphemisms which result in the patient making their own diagnosis by having to ask if you mean that they have cancer.
- Use pauses and body language to acknowledge they will need a moment to let the diagnosis sink in.
- Enquire if they have anyone with them to support them; they won't in the exam but it is good practice in the clinical setting.
- Ensure you've given contact details at the end of the consultation in case they think of more questions.

Module 14: Urogynaecology and Pelvic Floor Problems

It is expected that as an ST5 you would have a clear understanding of the anatomy, physiology and pathology of the pelvic floor and lower urinary tract. In addition, you should be able to take a full urogynaecological history, interpret routine investigations including urodynamics and understand the management of most urogynaecological conditions, even if you do not yet have the surgical skills to undertake many procedures. You should, however, have at least observed the majority of urogynaecological procedures.

While this module is primarily based around urogynaecology, a review of the core curriculum should remind you that it also includes faecal incontinence and treatment of acute bladder voiding disorders. It can be seen that there is a possible overlap in these areas of the core curriculum with the puerperium (module 8) and post-operative care (module 6). Thus, the final exam may not have 14 'pure' tasks, but could be composed of some which overlap two or more modules of the curriculum.

This module can easily be used to assess all five domains; however, it particularly lends itself to examining information gathering, communication with patients, patient safety and applied clinical knowledge, depending on how the task is constructed.

A typical task is shown below.

Candidate's Instructions

This is a simulated patient task covering:

- *information gathering*
- *communication with patients*
- *patient safety*
- *applied clinical knowledge.*

   You are an ST5 in the gynaecology clinic. Your next patient has attended for a routine follow-up six weeks after surgery. The case notes are missing, but the clinic staff have printed her discharge summary following her operation.

St. Paul's Hospital
Wood Lane
London
NW1 0SF

Discharge Summary

Re: Susie McDonald

Diagnosis:	*Stress incontinence*
Co-morbidity:	*Diabetes*
Operation:	*Tension free vaginal tape 25/4/16 by Mr Jackson*
Clinical course:	*Unremarkable.*
Fit note:	*2 weeks, no heavy lifting 6 weeks*
Analgesia:	*Patient's own*

Dr Bloomhead

Foundation doctor

   Ms McDonald has made a good recovery, but on examination you find a 5 mm diameter area of mesh exposed in the midline of the vagina suburethrally, at the site of the incision.

   You have ten minutes in which you should:

- *complete the history*
- *make a management plan*
- *answer the patient's questions*

Simulated Patient's Instructions

You are Susie McDonald, a 51-year-old secretary. You have three children, all normal deliveries, weighing 3.9 kg, 3.7 kg and 4.4 kg.

You became diabetic nine years ago, but this is generally well controlled with diet and metformin. Your last period was three years ago. You haven't been troubled by menopausal symptoms so didn't take hormone replacement.

Over the last few years you have been increasingly troubled by leakage of urine when you coughed, sneezed, laughed or tripped.

You saw the physiotherapists who taught you pelvic floor exercises, but these did not really help; then you saw a gynaecologist. After an uncomfortable bladder test they carried out what they called a tape procedure.

You are happy with the result of the operation. You no longer leak when you cough and sneeze. You no longer have any urinary problems: you don't have to rush to the toilet and you don't get up at night. As far as you are concerned the operation has been a complete success.

You had previously separated from your husband, but have started a new relationship this year. You think you may start to sleep together soon, which is partly what prompted you to get on with having surgery.

You have had no other surgery. You are on no other medication.

If not covered by the candidate, you could ask the following questions:

- *Why has this piece of tape become exposed?*
- *Do I have to have another operation? It feels fine now.*
- *Will cutting out some tape make me start leaking again?*
- *Can you check in my notes whether there was a problem during the operation which has caused this?*

Acting requirements:

- *If there has been no mention of tape erosion by midway through the task, you should ask: 'Was everything fine when you examined me?'*
- *From being happy and grateful for the results of the operation, you are now worried and upset on hearing that there is a complication.*

Notes on Your Approach to the Task

Examiner's Notes

This question, while clearly assessing the urogynaecology module, could also examine core surgical skills as it assesses a candidate's ability to understand and explain post-operative complications.

It can clearly be seen that the key issue for the competent candidate is to recognise that the patient is unaware that the vaginal wound has not healed. The competent candidate will therefore first gather information to check how satisfied the patient is with the procedure by means of a directed history within the time allowed, which should explore her diabetic control around the time of the procedure, and whether or not she was aware of any antibiotics being given. Next, they should ascertain whether the patient is aware of any problems or complications. In addition, at a follow-up visit a competent candidate would be expected to explicitly seek symptoms suggestive of complications, such as urgency, frequency or voiding problems.

Following this, the competent candidate will need to inform the patient of the tape exposure, and cope with her distress. Therefore, as part of the assessment of communication with patients, a competent candidate would be expected to be open, sensitive, honest and reassuring in respect of her ongoing symptom relief, yet clear about the need to correct the exposure.

In offering treatment options, the competent candidate will explain to the patient in a sensitive but objective manner that, left untreated, the exposed tape could lead to recurrent infection, recurrent bleeding and discomfort with intercourse for both her and her partner. In acknowledging to her that diabetic control, post-menopausal status, infection and surgical technique could all have contributed to the exposure, the competent candidate will be applying their clinical knowledge to reduce these risks as much as possible before an attempt is made to either bury or excise the exposed tape.

In addressing patient safety, the competent candidate should offer reassurance to the patient that exposure of the tape through the vaginal epithelium, while unfortunate and no doubt frustrating to the patient, is not a life-threatening condition. Thus, advising topical oestrogen and optimisation of diabetic control pre-operatively, and antibiotics peri-operatively, will demonstrate a logical approach to patient safety, in an attempt to minimise the risks and need for further procedures. However, the choice of whether the exposed tape is excised or over-sewn would be beyond the level of an ST5, although both options could be discussed.

The competent candidate, having assessed the situation, will apply their clinical knowledge to explain to the patient the possible contributing factors to the tape exposure, namely the fact that the patient is post-menopausal and diabetic, both of which increase the risk. However, the competent candidate will also provide reassurance that the tape can be re-epithelialised, and in order to reduce the risks of further erosion pre-operative topical oestrogen will help. Thereafter, depending on the clinical findings, attempts will be made either to mobilise the vaginal epithelium and over-sew the exposed tape or, if this is not possible, the exposed tape may need to be excised, which will of course put at risk any symptomatic improvement the patient has achieved.

Reflection on the Task

Review the notes you made before reading the examiner's notes. Did you understand that the patient is unaware of the exposed tape as this is a routine follow-up appointment rather than re-referral to clinic via the GP?

- This includes elements of breaking bad news as she has a complication which needs to be managed.
- Duty of candour requires an apology and explanation.
- You need to be able to discuss the management options while acknowledging that final decisions about the best approach would be taken at consultant level.

Summary

This chapter has provided you with an example of a task for each of the 14 modules tested in the Part 3 exam. By working through each example and referring to both the core curriculum and Part 3 assessment template, you should have developed a clear understanding of what will be assessed and the level of knowledge and skills you are expected to attain in order to achieve a pass. By providing you with the examiner's instructions and reflective notes, you should have gained a better understanding of how to approach each task and how to ensure that you pass each domain. There is no substitute for core knowledge, but learning how to approach a task will improve your chances of passing the exam and being awarded the MRCOG.

4 Tips for Candidates

This chapter is full of tips on preparing for an oral clinical examination. Many of the skills, in particular communication skills, required to pass the Part 3 exam need practice, so if you are reading this before sitting the written papers – well done! This gives you lots of time to prepare.

Usually, candidates will take up to six months to prepare for such important exams, so you need to develop a long-term strategy for passing the Part 3 exam. Your friends and family are essential in this process. They will provide you with support, reassurance and also with other activities to allow you time to relax and refresh so that you return to your studies with renewed enthusiasm.

If you are reading this having passed the Part 2 written exam, you've demonstrated that you have the knowledge required to meet the standards expected by the RCOG and now all you have to do is demonstrate your clinical skills to the examiners. Now you need to make a decision. Do you proceed to the Part 3 while the knowledge is fresh in your mind, or do you wait and prepare more fully for the clinical part of the exam? Ultimately the decision is yours, but we hope this chapter will help you decide what is right for you.

Don't Panic!

Every day in your routine clinical practice you are applying your clinical knowledge and thinking about patient safety in every decision you make. You are talking to patients and colleagues and gathering information as numerous clinical scenarios develop either slowly, such as in the outpatient setting, or rapidly, as in urgent care in obstetrics and gynaecology. These are the skills that will be assessed in the Part 3 examination, so if you are using these skills on a daily basis you should have no problem in passing the exam.

The MRCOG examination is aimed at the level of an ST5 trainee. You aren't expected to be an expert yet. An important aspect of patient safety is knowing when to call for help, and in some tasks you may fail if you don't inform your consultant just as you normally would in clinical practice. Calling for senior support is not a sign of lack of confidence or uncertainty about how to manage a problem. Equally, if you say you would 'call the consultant' for everything, that too could be wrong as you should be able to manage many things. The key is to make sure you seek help appropriately.

If you can view the examination as a normal day in antenatal clinic, gynaecology clinic, labour ward or being on call for emergencies, it will appear less daunting. Underpinning all of the clinical scenarios in the 14 tasks is an understanding of how obstetrics and gynaecology is practised in the NHS in the UK. For many trainees, both in the UK and overseas, the 'back office' functions of the NHS remain a mystery. It is essential that you understand how clinical governance shapes modern medical practice in terms of evidence-based practice, guidelines, incident reporting, audit and investigation of serious untoward events. It is also essential to understand the role of midwives, specialist nurses, the multidisciplinary team and allied health professionals working with doctors to provide a holistic approach to each patient's individual needs.

In summary, take a deep breath before you start each task and think to yourself: how would I approach this situation in my routine daily practice? Show the examiner that you are kind, caring, interested in your patient's concerns and that you can apply the knowledge that got you through the written papers.

Read the Question

This seems such basic advice but this really is very important. If a task asks you to:

- take a relevant history
- manage the immediate situation and
- make a management plan

then you are unlikely to pass if you spend all ten minutes just taking a history. This is a postgraduate exam so the examiners will be expecting a degree of sophistication in your clinical skills and will expect that you can manage your time to be able to address all of the requirements of the task. Remember, you do the same thing in every clinic to make sure all the patients are seen on time.

You are given two minutes to read the scenario before each task starts. The first time you read through the information posted on the outside of the booth, you will be focusing on the clinical material and searching through your memory banks for the relevant clinical knowledge, which is entirely reasonable. However, there is value in being more prepared than just focusing on the clinical basis for the task.

After you've considered the clinical setting for the task, go back and re-read the information again, but this time be more strategic and look for the clues hidden in the question. There will be key words or phrases which guide you as to how the marks will be awarded. Words like 'explain' or 'justify' are signposts to the skills that you are expected to demonstrate. If you develop a perfectly safe management plan but don't explain why you are suggesting this, or justifying why this is the preferred option, you are unlikely to pass.

Not all the clues are 'hidden'. Once you have read the clinical scenario, go back and look at what you have to do and the module and domains the task is assessing to decide on your strategic approach to the question.

Other clues are the 'hidden agenda' in a task. A task relating to a serious untoward event will award marks for dealing with the immediate issues, but a candidate is unlikely to pass if they don't also discuss the risk management issues arising from the situation. If a scenario seems very common and straightforward, there is likely to be a twist. Think about why this question is being included in the exam. For example, in a task focusing on pre-eclampsia, will the scenario evolve to become eclampsia or HELLP syndrome? If this is a problem in early pregnancy what are the less common features that could be explored in the task? In the next two chapters you will find further examples of how to strategically approach a task to understand where credit will be given.

Body Language

You've read the candidate information and the buzzer has sounded, so take a deep breath, think about your body language and step into the booth. In a structured discussion you are not expected to introduce yourself to the examiner, so just smile, say hello and sit down. The examiner will guide you into the start of the task.

If this is a task with a simulated patient, you need to adopt a friendly approach. This includes introducing yourself by name and checking how the patient would like to be addressed – for example, can you call her by her first name? Think carefully about your non-verbal communication; in most situations a friendly smile is appropriate, but if it's clear you are going to be breaking bad news a smile would be wrong, so show your sensitivity from the very beginning of the scenario.

Listen to the Actor's Questions

The actor may be in the role of a simulated patient or a simulated clinical colleague such as a nurse, midwife or junior doctor. The actor will have been carefully briefed about the scenario and will have some structured questions to ask you. These questions are designed to guide you so that you understand what you need to address in order to pass each domain.

In short, if the actor asks a question, listen carefully and then answer the question, the actor is trying to help you and won't be taking the discussion into an irrelevant area. In particular, if the actor asks the same question twice, be very careful to think about what you are doing or saying; they are trying to warn you that you are missing the point and trying to help you get back on track.

Another reason for questions is to try to move you on so that you have a chance to address all of their concerns and therefore achieve a pass. In summary, if the actor asks a question, listen carefully because they are trying to help you pass.

If There are Props, Use Them

There is likely to be some equipment on the table at one or more tasks on the exam circuit. This is particularly likely in a teaching task, where you might expect to find a doll and model of a pelvis for teaching breech delivery, for example. If there are props there, use them! The examiner will be expecting you to use the equipment to illustrate the points you are making.

Even more importantly, if this is a teaching task with a simulated junior doctor, ensure that they also use the props. Unless they have a chance to handle the props and show you what you have just taught them, you are unlikely to pass that domain.

It is, of course, imperative that you use the props correctly, so ensure that you are familiar with the standard equipment in everyday use in obstetrics and gynaecology. If you are working in a setting that, for example, doesn't have Kiwi® cups for ventouse delivery or Mirena IUS® for managing menorrhagia, ensure that you have used the resources on the RCOG website such as StratOG and other internet resources to fill the gaps in your knowledge.

Drawings

At the start of the examination, you will be given a notepad and pencil to take with you around the circuit. This is for you to take notes, but in reality is more of a 'comfort blanket' as you are unlikely to need to take extensive notes during the exam.

There is always debate about whether or not you should use drawings as part of your interaction with the simulated patient, and there is no definitive answer to this. The best advice would be to do whatever you do in normal everyday practice. If you routinely use a diagram to discuss, for example, the difference between a normal fallopian tube and a hydrosalpinx, then you will be good at doing these drawings; they will only take a couple of seconds and the interaction will feel natural. Some things are very difficult to represent pictorially and candidates will not fail a task for not including a drawing. Only use drawings if these really are a part of your routine practice and if you feel it will help explain something. Don't feel that you have to use a drawing for every situation as this isn't natural, will raise your stress levels and will interrupt the flow of the discussion.

Don't Point to Yourself

You should use the time preparing for the examination to look at your unconscious behaviours. It's very tempting to point to parts of your own body when trying to find out where a patient has pain or where you are going to make an incision, but this isn't to be recommended. If you point to yourself the person opposite will inevitably look where you are pointing and some patients (and examiners) may find this embarrassing.

Try to use words to describe the area you are referring to. For example, when describing the incision for a caesarean section, rather than pointing to your lower abdomen, explain that it will be just above the bikini line.

Euphemisms

In obstetrics and gynaecology we use strict anatomical terms when communicating with colleagues to ensure accurate communication; however, in the vast majority of discussions with patients we use alternative terms to describe parts of the body. It's very reasonable to use the word 'womb' instead of uterus when speaking to patients. When it comes to discussing genitalia it's much more difficult, and terms in common use in the English language can vary considerably. Depending on where the patient comes from in the UK, the vulva might be called any number of colloquial names, the commonest of which is 'down below'.

The safest approach is to find a term that you are comfortable with and that doesn't cause you embarrassment. When speaking to the patient, use the medical term (e.g. labia), and then explain in plain language (e.g. inner/outer lips) and then check that the patient has understood what you are referring to. Remember, you will be marked on whether you are able to communicate clearly with the patient in a way she understands, not on the words you use.

Resilience

The Part 3 exam is hard work. It is almost three hours long and there are no gaps or rest breaks, so it will be similar to one of your busiest days on call, with no coffee or comfort breaks, so you need to be prepared for this. This advice may seem really trivial, but in reality small problems can seriously affect a candidate's performance on the day. Make sure you have a good night's sleep the night before the exam. Consider staying overnight close to the exam centre rather than relying on long-distance travel early on the morning of the examination.

Don't panic and try to cram in last-minute revision on the morning of the exam. Last-minute revision never sticks in the memory and the Part 3 exam is all about core clinical skills rather than clinical minutiae.

Ensure you aren't overly tired on the day of the exam. Try to swap on-call commitments so that you aren't sitting the exam immediately after a weekend or series of nights on call. Don't stay up late the night before the Part 3 exam doing last-minute revision; remind yourself that you already have the required knowledge because you passed the Part 2 exam.

Have a proper breakfast/lunch before the exam (yes, this sounds like your parents talking) so that you don't lose concentration due to low blood sugar levels three-quarters of the way round the circuit. There are no rest breaks so no chances to top up declining blood glucose levels. Stay hydrated but don't drink so much that you need a comfort break during the exam circuit as you won't be given extra time if you need to leave the exam. Water will be available on the exam circuit.

Finally, you need to be comfortable during the exam so think about your appearance. This isn't a fashion show, but you are expected to present a professional appearance. Chose clothes and shoes that are comfortable, that fit well and that convey a professional, modest persona. It isn't essential to wear a suit, but casual wear would be inappropriate. Don't spend lots of money on new clothes and shoes, just make sure you are wearing something conservative and comfortable. Doctors in the UK have not worn white coats for several years, so there is no need to bring one.

Practice: Find an Exam Buddy

It is always easier to study for an exam if you can work with other people. You can share the tasks of summarising guidelines and making revision notes and you will probably have worked in a small group when preparing for the written exams. It is daunting to rehearse exam skills with people that you know, but if you work together you will both be able to reduce stress on the day of the exam and perform to your highest standard. If you can't bring yourself to rehearse with someone else, then practise out-loud in front of the mirror. Practise introducing yourself and giving your friendly smile. Use the scenarios in Chapters 3 and 5, set a timer for ten minutes and attempt the task verbally rather than mentally rehearsing. This will really help improve your exam skills.

Courses

It can be really helpful to attend a course in preparation for the Part 3 exam. Courses can help by demonstrating what a circuit feels like rather than practising tasks individually. The ability to move from task to task, and the resilience to not allow poor performance in one task to adversely affect the next task is a key exam skill. Use part of the initial two minutes' reading time of the next task to take a deep breath, clear your mind and focus, rather than concentrating on what you should or could have done better/differently in the last task. A mock circuit also helps to develop time management skills and stamina. It also helps to have an experienced trainer to advise you on your unconscious behaviours and polish your communication skills.

The best course to attend is the RCOG Part 3 preparatory course, as the faculty are trained and experienced examiners. They will therefore coach you in the relevant skills and attitudes that will be assessed in the real exam.

Look After Yourself

It takes at least six months to prepare for a postgraduate exam, and you will be working hard throughout that time in your evenings and weekends in addition to your clinical work. There is a lot of material to revise, including RCOG Green-top Guidelines, NICE guidelines and TOG articles, and achieving this in less than six months is challenging. If you decide to take the Part 3 immediately after the Part 2, make sure you have a break from revising before you start the final preparation for Part 3.

During the preparation time it's really important to stay healthy. Make sure you take some exercise on a regular basis and that you have a healthy diet. Avoid cramming for the exam by using stimulants like caffeine to keep you awake and revising into the early hours of the morning. Your sleep is an important part of learning and memory. Rapid eye movement (REM) sleep allows facts to be stored in long-term memory and REM sleep is disturbed by the use of stimulants.

Don't neglect your friends and family. It's important for everyone to maintain a work–life balance and this principle also applies to exams. There is good evidence that concentration decreases after approximately 40 minutes of study, so taking a break to catch up with a friend, have something to eat or drink or phone home will help. You can then return to your studies and you will find that you can concentrate again. It is a hard time but it doesn't last forever.

It is recommended that you attempt the Part 3 exam straight after passing the Part 2 exam so that you can make the best use of all those months of revision. Leaving a long gap between Part 2 and Part 3 means you will have to go back and re-revise all those topics again.

Finally, make sure this really is the right time for you to attempt the exams. For candidates in the UK specialty training programme, there is obviously pressure to have passed the exams by the end of your ST5 year so that you can progress to higher training, but life also happens in the meantime, including stressful life events such as moving house, having babies or illness of family members. If you have other pressures in your life, think about postponing the exam until those stresses are resolved and you can focus on your studies. Remember, you can also put a lot of pressure on yourself if you attempt the exam too early in your career.

5   Practice Tasks with Videos

Task 1: Meconium Stained Liquor (Simulated Patient Task)

This task relates to module 6, management of labour (core curriculum module 10).

Candidate's Instructions

This is a simulated patient task assessing:

- *information gathering*
- *patient safety*
- *communication with patients*
- *applied clinical knowledge.*

You are the ST5 on call for the Obstetric Unit and have been asked to review Mary Bold, who is a patient in the Midwifery-Led Unit downstairs. She is a primigravida at 41 weeks' gestation who presented earlier this morning in spontaneous labour.

She had spontaneous rupture of her membranes ten hours ago and was 3 cm dilated at that stage. She is contracting 2–3:10 minutes and the contractions are lasting 20 seconds. Fresh meconium has been identified and the midwife has confirmed that the lie is longitudinal with a cephalic presentation, the head being 2/5 palpable. A vaginal examination shows that the cervix is still 3 cm dilated, fully effaced with the head 1 cm above the spines with caput +. The midwife has asked you to review the case and agree a management plan with Mary.

You have ten minutes in which you should:

- *establish the full extent of the situation, including the patient's wishes*
- *manage the immediate situation and agree a plan for the labour*
- *advise on the next steps to be taken*

Spend two minutes thinking about how you would approach this task, making notes if it helps you. Think about how you would approach this situation; what communication skills do you need? Consider how you would establish a rapport with the patient and identify her concerns and respect her autonomy. Then watch the two videos linked to the task. Make notes about the performance of the actor playing the role of the candidate in the core clinical skills that are being assessed in this task. For each of the clinical skills, decide if the candidate's skills are at the level of a pass, fail or borderline.

After you have watched and scored this task you can compare your assessment with the comments of trained Part 3 clinical and lay examiners. The aim of this process is to show you what behaviours are expected and to understand how you will be marked when you attempt the Part 3 examination.

Task 1, video 1: videos are hosted at www.cambridge.org/9781316627457

Video 1: Your Clinical Examiner Comments

Information Gathering

Comments:

Pass   Borderline   Fail

Communication with Patients

Comments:

Pass   Borderline   Fail

Patient Safety

Comments:

Pass   Borderline   Fail

Applied Clinical Knowledge

Comments:

      Pass   Borderline   Fail

Now compare your comments and decisions with those of the clinical and lay examiners.

Video 1: Clinical Examiner Comments

Information Gathering

> Comments:
>
> • *Quickly established facts, used open questions, ascertains reasons for concern, good signposting of discussion, explains terminology - meconium.*

(Pass)   Borderline   Fail

Communication with Patients

> Comments:
>
> • *Introduced herself with name and role, explained why she had been called. Good body language, empathic and actively listening, pauses to allow patient to breathe through contraction, respects her views, gave reassurance. Acknowledged concerns.*
> • *'Nothing without your consent.'*
> • *Personalises discussion, checks it's OK to carry on after contraction.*

(Pass)   Borderline   Fail

Patient Safety

> Comments:
>
> • *Offers rather than instructs increased monitoring by CTG, explains need to inform consultant, gives clear reason for not using pool, explains latent phase and significance of lack of progress, respects patient's concerns and autonomy, maintains patient dignity through non-verbal and verbal skills.*

(Pass)   Borderline   Fail

Applied Clinical Knowledge

> Comments:
>
> • *Synthesises a management plan - repeat VE in four hours? Offers telemetry and explains why need CTG. Needs to be clearer about risks.*

Pass   (Borderline)   Fail

Video 1: Lay Examiner Comments

Information Gathering

> **Comments:**
>
> - *Finds out patient's wishes, gives patient time to think things through - not rushed into decision, is very calm and reassuring. Addresses concerns about bonding and wanting natural birth. 'Try to keep things as natural as you can.'*
> - *Doesn't alarm the patient at all. Finds out the patient wants to wait for her husband, takes time to find out his name and uses it to make conversation more personal.*

        Borderline   Fail

Communication with Patients

> **Comments:**
>
> - *Compassionate, empathic and addresses the patient's needs. Explains 'what we offer and why' - monitoring to listen to heartbeat to see if baby is in distress, explains need for transfer and what will happen in extremely understandable way. Hormone injection - how this will make things progress for her.*
> - *'Making decisions together', 'will be a joint decision as to what we do' - respect for patient's views, risks put across in a non-scary way and that things may happen as a possibility, not that they will happen if she doesn't transfer. Comes to mutually agreed plan - shared decision making - crucial.*

        Borderline   Fail

Before you watch video 2, you may find it helpful to read the instructions given to the simulated patient. They are given detailed instructions so that their performance is consistent throughout the exam, ensuring that each candidate has the same opportunity to pass the task in all the areas assessed. The actor is given guidance about how the competent candidate will tackle the task. This may give you an insight into how the actor tries to help candidates by prompting them and asking questions. However, it is very important to remember that the actor is allowed to react to what the candidate is saying so may become upset or angry if the candidate says or does something that is ill-advised. The actor won't shout or swear though.

Simulated Patient's Instructions

You are Mary Bold, a 39-year-old solicitor in your first pregnancy. You are 41 weeks pregnant and there have been no problems during the pregnancy. You and your partner Liam have researched labour and are very keen for minimal intervention. You are very much of the view that nature is best and that doctors often intervene and create problems in so doing.

You are happy for intermittent monitoring of the baby's heartbeat but do not want continuous CTG monitoring. Ideally you want a water birth in the Midwifery-Led Unit and cannot see why with a straightforward pregnancy this cannot be possible.

The thought of an epidural and being connected to a drip is your worst-case scenario. You are concerned that this could affect bonding with your baby and breastfeeding. Overall the health of your baby is very important to you, so if sensible proposals are explained to you then you will be flexible in the interests of your baby.

You will not accept a proposed management plan that would entail transfer to the Consultant-Led Labour Ward for continuous CTG monitoring and augmentation with Syntocinon®, but would agree to a compromise such as transfer to the labour ward and CTG monitoring alone.

The competent candidate will:

- *quickly elicit a history and establish the nature of the problem*
- *explain the situation and rationale of the proposed management plan to you*
- *advise of the need to transfer you to the labour ward for additional care*
- *advise of the risks if you don't agree with the management plan and work with you to reach a compromise*
- *emphasise the need for increased monitoring and the need to involve the consultant in your care*
- *negotiate a management plan to keep you and your baby as safe as possible*

Now watch video 2 and score the candidate. How does their performance differ from video 1? Also consider how similar the approach is by the actor to each of the candidates.

Task 1, video 2: videos are hosted at www.cambridge.org/9781316627457

Video 2: Your Clinical Examiner Comments
Information Gathering

Comments:

Pass   Borderline   Fail

Communication with Patients

Comments:

Pass   Borderline   Fail

Patient Safety

Comments:

Pass   Borderline   Fail

Applied Clinical Knowledge

Comments:

Pass   Borderline   Fail

Now compare your comments and decisions with those of the clinical and lay examiners.

Video 2: Clinical Examiner Comments

Information Gathering

Comments:

- Limited information gathering, straight into plan. Did use open questions but didn't gather information about the patient's wishes.

Pass   Borderline   Fail

Communication with Patients

Comments:

- Good eye contact but didn't introduce herself by name or role. Active listening but no empathy, clearly under pressure so carries on talking during contraction to get her point across.
- Interrupts patient, doesn't respect her views: 'listen to me for a second'. Talks about costs and benefits, not patient's agenda.
- Uses jargon to intimidate patient: meconium - 'faeces'.

Pass   Borderline   Fail

Patient Safety

Comments:

- Recognises risks of fetal distress, mentions brain damage but in a way that is coercing patient by trying to frighten her.
- Labour ward 'safe environment' - implies Midwifery-Led Unit isn't safe - undermining colleagues.
- 'You won't have a normal birth' - recognises could need caesarean section but does not respect the patient's right to make decisions against medical advice. Doesn't suggest involving a consultant.

Pass   Borderline   Fail

Applied Clinical Knowledge

Comments:

- Recognises the significance of meconium - distress, meconium aspiration syndrome.
- Understands cannot determine variability by auscultation.
- Plan to move to labour ward, site epidural and start Syntocinon® is appropriate, but takes no account of patient's wishes - epidural is stated, not offered.

Pass   (Borderline)   Fail

Video 2: Lay Examiner Comments

Information Gathering

> Comments:
>
> - *Doesn't check understanding of the patient at all, doesn't summarise and doesn't recognise that the patient wants a water birth with no intervention.*
> - *Doesn't ask the right questions.*

Pass   Borderline   Fail

Communication with Patients

> Comments:
>
> - *Ignores the patient's comments regarding breastfeeding and bonding. Doesn't involve the partner - 'you have to go to labour ward now'. Terms - meconium, Syntocinon® - technical terms, doesn't say what it is, how it might affect the baby or why it is important. Bullying the patient, very threatening.*
> - *Keeps saying things are very serious, alarming the patient. Doesn't listen to the patient or ask what she wants. Doesn't answer the patient's question about implications of not agreeing to the plan: 'Will my baby die?'*

Pass   Borderline   Fail

Review the notes that you made before you started to watch the videos and compare your judgement with that of the clinical and lay examiners. Did you agree with them? Was there anything else you would have done in the task to negotiate an agreed management plan with this patient? Do you have a clear understanding of why the candidates were given their scores and what they could have done to improve?

It might help you to understand the examiner's assessments if you read through their instructions.

Clinical Examiner's Instructions

Familiarise yourself with the candidate's instructions and role player's information sheet. Agree an approach to the assessment with the lay examiner.

The competent candidate will establish the purpose of the consultation and the midwife's concerns. A relevant obstetric history will be taken, and Ms Bold's views on labour and delivery will be ascertained.

The competent candidate will explain to Ms Bold that the current situation may be placing her baby at increased risk and so action may be necessary in order to prevent harm. The increased risks with fresh meconium in labour will be discussed, with an examination offered and a recommendation made for continuous CTG monitoring in an obstetric labour ward unit. The lack of progress in labour will be recognised, and augmentation with Syntocinon® advised.

The competent candidate will adopt a non-threatening style, acknowledging the patient's distress and frustration, and that this was not what she had planned for her labour experience. It will be reinforced that positive steps should be taken to reach a compromise and agree a management plan, with consultant input advised.

Reassurance will be provided that nothing will be done without the patient's consent, while ensuring that she appreciates the potential risks and implications of non-compliance.

Lay Examiner's Instructions

Familiarise yourself with the candidate's instructions and the simulated patient's instructions.

Score the candidate's performance on the results sheet.
The competent candidate will:

- *quickly elicit a history and establish the nature of the problem*
- *explain the situation and rationale of the proposed management plan to the patient*
- *emphasise the advice for increased monitoring and obstetric involvement in her care*
- *advise of a need for transfer to the obstetric labour ward for additional care*
- *advise of the risks if such a management plan is not agreed and work with the patient to reach an agreement*
- *'negotiate' a management plan to keep mother and baby as safe as possible*

Learning Points

The clinical knowledge on which this scenario is based is core knowledge. In everyday practice this situation of slow progress in labour in a woman pregnant for the first time with meconium stained liquor is common and will be familiar to all ST5 trainees. In both cases, the candidates clearly understand the implications of the situation and both know what is expected in terms of the management plan, so they clearly both have the required level of knowledge to pass this task.

Watching the videos and reading the clinical and lay examiner's comments should explain why candidates with a similar level of knowledge can pass or fail purely due to their approach and professional attitudes.

Read the Question

It is very easy to spend the two minutes reading time focusing on the clinical scenario and making notes about what your management plan will be. While having the clinical knowledge and being able to synthesise and justify a management plan is essential, there are clues in the question about what else is needed to pass the task. What have you been asked to do?

1. **Establish the *full extent* of the situation, including the patient's *wishes***

The words 'full extent' should give you a clue that there is more to this scenario than managing primary arrest in labour with meconium. This should alert you to the need to ask open questions about the patient's concerns. The simulated patient will then share with you her desire for a natural birth with no intervention, her mistrust of doctors and her desire to wait until her husband is back before making a decision. The task clearly states that it will assess information gathering and communication with the patient, so in preparing for the task, the competent candidate will recognise the need to ask about 'her wishes' as well as her clinical background.

2. **Manage the immediate situation and *agree* a plan for the labour**

The use of the word 'agree' rather than 'decide on' should give you a clue that the simulated patient is likely to disagree with standard advice. The skills being tested are the ability to negotiate with a patient while ensuring you keep her and her baby safe. This involves being able to establish a rapport with the patient and deal with her reluctance to accept your advice without the situation developing into anger or an argument. In negotiations, each side has to compromise a little in order to meet in the middle. The actor has been briefed to agree to a compromise if approached correctly. The task clearly states that patient safety will be assessed. It is important to distinguish between a compromise that retains elements of patient safety and collusion with a patient's request that puts her or her baby at risk. The skill lies in being able to point out in a non-threatening way that her first request for no intervention is no longer a safe option.

3. ***Advise* on the next steps to be taken**

The use of the word 'advise' should alert you to the need to make a plan without confrontation. This is not the same as simply telling the patient what must be done. This implies that you need to be able to justify and explain the reasons behind your suggestions. The task states that applied clinical knowledge is being assessed and the ability to explain the clinical evidence that supports your management plan is an essential skill.

Summary

Each task will assess between three and five core clinical skills, so knowledge alone will not be sufficient to pass the Part 3 exam. It is an important part of examination technique to look for the key words in the instructions to help plan your approach and to utilise the skills that have been defined in Chapter 2 and on the RCOG website.

Task 2: Tutorial on Electrosurgery (Structured Discussion Task)

This task relates to module 2, core surgical skills (module 5 of the core curriculum), but could equally be used to assess module 1, teaching.

Candidate's Instructions

This task is a structured discussion assessing:

- *communication with colleagues*
- *patient safety*
- *applied clinical knowledge.*

   The case of Mrs Joyce Adams was discussed at the monthly Governance Meeting. Mrs Adams is a 48-year-old midwife who sustained a bowel injury after elective surgery performed by her consultant. The injury was diagnosed ten days after a laparoscopic left salpingo-oophorectomy to remove a large dermoid cyst. The left ovary was adherent to the sigmoid colon and the operating surgeon used a combination of monopolar and bipolar diathermy to free the ovary. The meeting concluded that the perforation had occurred as a result of thermal damage to the sigmoid colon.

   As part of the action plan, you (as an ST5) have been asked to organise a feedback session on electrosurgery. This will involve all grades of doctors in the department as well as theatre staff. Your task is to explain the background to the session and the possible mechanisms of electrosurgical damage, and to cover the basic principles of monopolar diathermy, in particular highlighting how problems can arise. You are about to explain to the Clinical Lead for Governance how you plan to approach the session. The Clinical Lead has been asked not to interrupt you over the allocated time.

   You have ten minutes in which you should:

- *refer to the index case*
- *cover the basic principles of electrosurgery*
- *highlight how problems occur and how to avoid them*
- *make reference to the items provided by way of illustration*

[NOTE – equipment provided: an electrosurgical generator, a monopolar pad with lead attached, a selection of instruments including graspers, scissors and bipolar forceps with lead attached, a selection of plastic and metal trocars.]

   Spend two minutes thinking about how you would approach this task, making notes if it helps you. Then watch the two videos linked to the task. Make notes about the performance of the actor playing the role of the candidate in the core clinical skills that are being assessed in this task. For each of the clinical skills, decide whether the candidate's skills are at the level of a pass, fail or borderline.

After you have watched and scored this task you can compare your assessment with the comments of a trained Part 3 examiner. The aim of this process is to show you what behaviours are expected and to understand how you will be marked when you attempt the Part 3 exam.

Task 2, video 1: videos are hosted at www.cambridge.org/9781316627457

Video 1: Your Clinical Examiner Comments

Communication with Colleagues

```
Comments:




```

Pass   Borderline   Fail

Patient Safety

```
Comments:




```

Pass   Borderline   Fail

Applied Clinical Knowledge

```
Comments:




```

Pass   Borderline   Fail

Now compare your comments and decisions with those of the clinical examiner

Video 1: Clinical Examiner Comments

Communication with Colleagues

> Comments:
>
> - *Clearly understands reasons for the session in terms of avoidable injury, has reviewed the case, recognises the need to involve all theatre staff as well as junior doctors and consultants.*
> - *Shows understanding of the need to tackle difficult issues with colleagues - experience of the consultant, using wrong hands, Hassan entry, use of monopolar diathermy close to the bowel.*
> - *Logical and coherent approach to the tutorial, good use of props. Clear plan for the tutorial.*

(Pass)   Borderline   Fail

Patient Safety

> Comments:
>
> - *Appreciates the difference between bipolar and monopolar - safety, spread of thermal damage. Demonstrates clear understanding of equipment provided. Risk factors are identified - exit burns from monopolar pad, metal trocars, machine settings, foot peddle in reach. Notes the need to maintain visual field.*
> - *Need to call for help, general surgeons, urogynaecologist.*
> - *Checking in - identifying any implants, team debrief.*
> - *Need to incident report when re-admitted.*

(Pass)   Borderline   Fail

Applied Clinical Knowledge

> Comments:
>
> - *Clear understanding of the clinical implications of the topic. Understands mechanism of injury.*
> - *WHO checklist, team work, use of assistant. Avoid electrosurgery near the bowel.*
> - *Justifies equipment choice and options.*
> - *Can clearly work under pressure.*

(Pass)   Borderline   Fail

Did you agree with the clinical examiner's assessment of the candidate? Are there any significant gaps in knowledge or patient safety? Would you have chosen a similar approach to the structure, content and audience for the tutorial?

Before you watch the next video it may help to read the examiner's instructions.

Video 1: Examiner's Instructions

The competent candidate will establish the purpose of the session and why it is required.

The competent candidate should be able to talk openly to the Governance Lead as to the likely cause of the injury.

The competent candidate should explain that this situation should not have occurred and is most likely linked to mobilisation of the ovary.

They should be able to explain the principal of monopolar diathermy (in which the current passes from the generator through an active electrode – scissors/grasper – then through the tissues and back to the return plate and away from the patient). They should be able to differentiate between cut and coagulation currents.

They should be able to explain that bipolar diathermy does not require the patient to complete the circuit and that current passes from one side of the electrode to the other, just affecting the tissue in between that is being treated and is therefore safer.

The competent candidate should be able to discuss the risks of diathermy to include direct and indirect burns and potential issues such as surgical smoke.

They should have an understanding that there are different power settings, and different instruments will have different current densities associated with their use.

The candidate should demonstrate an ability to teach objectively using the scenario as an example, not mentioning specific details of the patient, and will support their talk with reference to the props provided.

Now watch video 2 and make notes on the candidate's performance.
Task 2, video 2: videos are hosted at www.cambridge.org/9781316627457

Video 2: Your Clinical Examiner Comments

Communication with Colleagues

Comments:

Pass   Borderline   Fail

Patient Safety

Comments:

Pass   Borderline   Fail

Applied Clinical Knowledge

Comments:

Pass   Borderline   Fail

Again, compare your comments and decisions with those of the clinical examiner.

Video 2: Clinical Examiner Comments

Communication with Colleagues

> Comments:
> - *Clearly hasn't read the scenario - assumes a consultant didn't do the case. Fails to recognise that the whole team needs to be involved in a training session not just registrars - plans not to involve consultants or very junior doctors.*
> - *Didn't recognise that this was a delayed thermal injury so wouldn't have been recognised at the time of operation.*
> - *Hasn't included theatre nurses in the plan - ?blaming nurses for not putting diathermy pad on correctly.*

Pass   Borderline

Patient Safety

> Comments:
> - *Hasn't described adverse incident reporting process.*
> - *Doesn't acknowledge sub-standard care - appears to be apportioning blame.*
> - *Assumption that if the patient has given consent, they should accept the risk of an adverse event - comments that bowel injuries are 'common'.*
> - *Doesn't understand the mechanism of injury; misunderstanding about thermal spread of monopolar and bipolar.*
> - *Advises looking down at peddles before using diathermy; doesn't understand the risks.*

Pass   Borderline

Applied Clinical Knowledge

> Comments:
> - *Cardiac problems*
> - *Doesn't stimulate muscles and nerves*
> - *Understands cutting, coagulation and blend settings*
> - *Choice of monopolar or bipolar*
> - *Is able to demonstrate equipment*

Pass   Borderline   Fail

How closely do you agree with the clinical examiner in each case? Do you agree with their decision about passing and failing in each of the three clinical skills assessed? If necessary, re-watch the video to see why they made those comments. This should help you to understand how the clinical examiners make their assessments and what behaviours they are looking for.

Reflect on the notes that you made before you watched the videos, would you have used a similar approach to this task? Is there anything else you feel should have been included? Is there anything they did that you wouldn't have thought of?

Learning Points

The instructions for this task give the candidate a clear indication of the clinical skills being assessed and clear instructions about what they need to do.

Read the Question

1. Organise a feedback session on electrosurgery

This task focuses on the candidate's ability to make a plan to deliver a tutorial, which is an assessment of teaching skills. Core teaching skills require an understanding of the aims and objectives of a tutorial, the knowledge level of the attendees and a structured and comprehensive approach to the task. Before starting to create a PowerPoint presentation, an outline plan is essential and that is what is required for this task.

2. Explain ... how you *plan* to approach the session

The candidate needs to discuss both 'what' and 'how'. It's very easy to concentrate on telling the examiner **what** you know about electrosurgery and fail to specify **how** you would set up the feedback session, who you would include, where the training should take place and how you would identify a suitable time to ensure good attendance. Remember who will need to be there. You will need to make sure the teaching is appropriate to all levels of staff and all professional groups.

3. Refer to the *index case*

The candidate's instructions make it clear that they are required to refer to the index case so the tutorial should be focused very specifically on use of diathermy at laparoscopic adhesiolysis involving the bowel. The instructions also make it clear that the candidate is expected to use the props provided to illustrate their tutorial. This is because a modern approach to medical education recognises the limitations of 'chalk and talk' as it is very common for the attendees to lose concentration and interest if they are being talked at rather than being involved in the session. A blended approach is more appropriate and use of equipment allows attendees to actively participate in the session, which will reinforce the learning points. The RCOG curriculum makes clear the need to understand modern teaching methods.

4. Cover the basic principles of electrosurgery

Another essential teaching skill is a detailed understanding of the topic that you are teaching so a clear understanding of the safe use of diathermy is essential to achieve a pass in the applied clinical knowledge domain.

5. Highlight *how* problems occur and how to avoid them

The task is not purely about testing the candidate's knowledge about diathermy; the subtlety of this task is that it also assesses an understanding of critical incident investigation, the need to develop an action plan after a root cause analysis of a critical incident and understanding that any action plan may need to include the wider team such as nurses, midwives and operating department practitioners.

A root cause analysis aims to identify a number of things. It will identify whether there are problems with one individual who may need training or support with a particular aspect of their clinical skills, or a systematic problem with processes relating to safe surgery. You should understand that this is not the same as blaming an individual for an adverse event. While the NHS and the GMC do require each individual to take responsibility for their clinical skills, the philosophy is one of learning from adverse events rather than apportioning blame. In tasks relating to adverse events you should take care to avoid apportioning blame. Thus, it is important to consider whether one experienced member of the team can cause an incident like this; a root cause analysis may well recognise that there is a risk that many members of the team may not understand the detailed issues related, in this case, to electrosurgery, and hence require a general update for all personnel.

The root cause analysis will also identify systems problems – for example, an organisational culture that doesn't implement safety measures such as the WHO safe surgery checklist – or equipment problems such as the lack of appropriate equipment – for example, the appropriate bipolar instruments to be used in dissection close to the bowel. The root cause analysis is not an exercise in apportioning blame; it is a mechanism to prevent further similar adverse events.

Summary

This is a further example of using examination technique to think strategically about your approach to a task. The two minutes of thinking time is the opportunity for you to concentrate on the specific words and phrases that are used to guide you about the skills being tested.

In a task like this it would be very easy just to talk to the examiner about electrosurgery rather than explaining 'how you would approach the session', and hopefully now you will realise why that will not be enough to achieve a pass. It is clear that you must have a good understanding of electrosurgery in order to pass this task; after all, you use diathermy every day in routine clinical practice. Understanding how a diathermy machine works is basic knowledge, which is tested in the Part 1 MRCOG exam, so it should be obvious that electrosurgery is just the framework in which to test more sophisticated skills, competencies and attitudes.

Task 3: Teaching Ventouse Delivery (Simulated Colleague Task)

This task relates to module 1 – teaching – part of core curriculum module 2 – teaching, appraisal and assessment – although it could also be used to assess module 7 – management of delivery.

Candidate's Instructions

This is a simulated trainee task assessing:

- *applied clinical knowledge*
- *communication with colleagues*
- *patient safety.*

As the ST5 on call for obstetrics and gynaecology, you have just delivered Lucy Brown using a ventouse and have been asked to teach the technique to a junior colleague with no prior experience of the procedure.

You have ten minutes to demonstrate how you would teach the technique of a Kiwi® vacuum delivery in a case such as this to a junior colleague with no prior experience of the procedure.

For this task, the instructions to the simulated junior colleague are very simple.

Simulated Trainee's Instructions

You are a junior doctor (ST1) with no prior experience of delivering a baby by vacuum extraction. You have asked the ST5 doctor (Registrar) on call with you today to teach you the procedure.
The ST5 doctor must explain the procedure to you in a clear and logical manner and allow you to handle the equipment and practise its use.

As you can see from these instructions, there are no tricks or traps in this task. The actor hasn't been instructed to do anything unpredictable or to get upset or angry. This is a straightforward task of teaching a practical skill.

Spend two minutes thinking about how you would approach this task, making notes if it helps you. Then watch the two videos of the candidates teaching the simulated junior trainee. For each of the clinical skills domains, decide whether the candidate's skills are at the level of a pass, fail or borderline.

After you have watched and scored this task you can compare your assessment with the comments of a trained Part 3 examiner. The aim of this process is to show you what behaviours are expected and to understand how you will be marked when you attempt the Part 3 exam.

Task 3, video 1: videos are hosted at www.cambridge.org/9781316627457

Video 1: Your Clinical Examiner Comments
Applied Clinical Knowledge

Comments:

Pass	Borderline	Fail

Communication with Colleagues

Comments:

Pass	Borderline	Fail

Patient Safety

Comments:

Pass	Borderline	Fail

Now compare your comments and decisions with those of the clinical examiner.

Video 1: Clinical Examiner Comments

Applied Clinical Knowledge

> Comments:
> - Clearly experienced in the technique of ventouse delivery, logical approach, correct sequence.
> - Explains the need for a catheter, how to guide the woman's pushing. Didn't mention asking mum to pant when head crowning.
> - Lack of detail about where to make the episiotomy, specified 45 degrees then 60 degrees.
> - Did specify gentle traction and calling for senior help or ultrasound scan if position not clear.

Pass　　　　　　　　　(Borderline)　　　　　　　　　Fail

Communication with Colleagues

> Comments:
> - Clear explanation of purpose and scope of the teaching session. Checks knowledge of the trainee; corrects VE technique 'use two fingers, whole hand will hurt'; shows how to pump up ventouse and then gives trainee chance to try it. Encourages trainee to be hands-on, talking throughout.
> - Correctly explains caput, moulding, OA position and station.

(Pass)　　　　　　　　　Borderline　　　　　　　　　Fail

Patient Safety

> Comments:
> - Emphasises need to introduce herself to mum and keep mum informed throughout delivery. Explains the need to do abdominal exam as well as VE. Checks for full dilatation and position. Cleans and drapes, local anaesthetic for episiotomy.
> - Explains nuchal cord, delivery of shoulders and cord gases.
> - Needed to be prompted to define flexion point.

(Pass)　　　　　　　　　Borderline　　　　　　　　　Fail

You can see in video 1 how the actor prompted the candidate to define the flexion point, a good example of how the actor uses questions to guide the candidate to a key skill that needs to be included in their tutorial.

Before you watch the second video, read the clinical examiner's instructions.

> **Clinical Examiner's Instructions**
>
> *Familiarise yourself with the candidate's instructions and simulated junior doctor's instructions. Plan your approach to the task together.*
>
> *You are to listen to the candidate's description of how to teach a junior colleague the technique employed to deliver Lucy Brown – the preparation, technique and precautions employed.*
>
> *The competent candidate will demonstrate correct positioning, the need to clean, drape and catheterise, and prior perineal infiltration with local anaesthetic in case of episiotomy.*
>
> *The procedure will be taught at each stage with reference to the patient's role in the delivery, including when to push and when to breathe.*
>
> *The competent candidate will emphasise the need for correct assessment of the position of the fetal head and note the clinical findings, including dilatation, position, station, caput and moulding.*
>
> *The demonstration will include how the equipment functions, including application of lubricant, correct application of the Kiwi® cup to the fetal head and correct application of pressure.*
>
> *The candidate will teach how to deliver the baby safely, in the correct direction, with appropriate dialogue with the patient at the correct times – when to push/breathe and stipulate when to abandon the procedure (after three pulls).*
>
> *The candidate will explain the assessment for episiotomy, safe removal of the cup, a check for the cord around the neck and allowing for restitution of the fetal head.*
>
> *The candidate will explain how the perineum and vagina are then assessed for lacerations, with repair as necessary. The blood loss will be estimated and medical records completed.*

You should note that in the real exam you wouldn't be permitted to carry on talking after the buzzer has sounded, the examiner will move you on to the next booth as they only have two minutes to document their assessment of your performance in each domain.

Now watch the second video and mark this candidate's teaching session in the three clinical skills domains.

Task 3, video 2: videos are hosted at www.cambridge.org/9781316627457

Video 2: Your Clinical Examiner Comments

Applied Clinical Knowledge

Comments:

Pass   Borderline   Fail

Communication with Colleagues

Comments:

Pass   Borderline   Fail

Patient Safety

Comments:

Pass   Borderline   Fail

Now compare your notes with those of the examiner. Did you agree on the marks?

Video 2: Clinical Examiner Comments

Applied Clinical Knowledge

> Comments:
>
> - *Can clearly do ventouse but didn't explain a logical approach. Advised to feel the abdomen and then get consent. Advises ventouse when station at spines. Tells her to feel for landmarks, but didn't explain.*
> - *Didn't clean and drape patient, didn't check for full dilatation.*

Pass   Borderline    Fail

Communication with Colleagues

> Comments:
>
> - *Starts by telling her off - you should have done some reading first.*
> - *Uses a lot of technical terms without explaining, just keeps asking 'is that clear?' Doesn't explain what and where re: episiotomy. Describes fontanelles but doesn't use doll to explain. Doesn't show her first, takes over rather than correcting technique.*
> - *Did manage time well and did ask what went well and what could have been better.*

Pass   (Borderline)   Fail

Patient Safety

> Comments:
>
> - *Description of instrumental delivery as painful and traumatising. Incorrect definition of flexion point, three attempts if the cup pops off, won't answer the question - 'that's too advanced'.*
> - *Prompted by actor about analgesia.*

Pass   Borderline   Fail

Did you agree with the examiner? You can see from the examiner's comments that the passing standard for this task is high. This is because the clinical scenario is a routine everyday situation and trainees should have mastered the technique of ventouse delivery at a much earlier stage than ST5, so errors in technique would be a serious cause for concern.

Why do you think we use an actor for a task like this rather than a real trainee? If we were to use a real trainee they would already know some of the steps in the procedure, whereas an actor is skilled in 'playing' a role of no knowledge over and over again.

However, before the exam the actor will have been properly trained by the examiners to perform a ventouse so they understand the prompts to give you so you have every opportunity to pass this task.

Learning Points

The ability to teach is an essential clinical skill as defined by both the Part 2 MRCOG curriculum and by the GMC in *Good Medical Practice*. In order to be able to teach a skill, the teacher must be at the top of Miller's triangle (Figure 5.1) for that skill and be competent in that skill. Assessing the skill of vacuum delivery should be straightforward for candidates attempting Part 3 as this method of delivery is in everyday use on the labour ward. If the only purpose of this task was to assess the ability to carry out a vacuum delivery, this could be easily assessed by workplace-based assessment, so it should be clear that this Part 3 task tests deeper skills than just the ability to carry out a vacuum delivery.

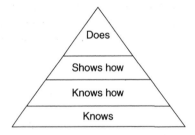

Figure 5.1 Miller's skills triangle.

Read the Question

1. **The task will assess . . . applied clinical knowledge**

The instructions clearly ask the candidate to relate the teaching '**to a case such as this**', which should indicate the need to be very specific about a vacuum Kiwi® delivery in the context of a ventouse delivery for failure to progress with a direct occipito-anterior position. Therefore a tutorial about instrumental delivery in general is unlikely to pass because even if the clinical knowledge is correct, it isn't being appropriately **applied** to this case. Similarly, any time spent discussing delivery of any baby that is not occipito-anterior is unlikely to gain you any credit, as it would be inappropriate to teach anything other than a direct occipito-anterior delivery to such a junior trainee.

As part of the teaching session, the competent candidate will spend just a couple of moments explaining why this is the correct choice of instrument in this case. The instructions make it very clear that this is to be a practical demonstration, so you shouldn't spend the whole time explaining the theory. In the second video we saw that the candidate didn't make good use of the props and didn't give the trainee much chance to be hands-on.

2. Communication with colleagues

Communication between medical colleagues requires a different skill from communication with patients. We use medical language to ensure that our communication is accurate and precise, and not open to misinterpretation. We therefore have to ensure that junior colleagues understand the language of medicine, so while we would expect to communicate using 'medical jargon', it is still just as important to check understanding. In the Part 3 exam it is a slightly artificial situation as the simulated junior colleagues are actors and therefore wouldn't understand anatomical terms as a real ST1 would, but you are using this as an opportunity to demonstrate your knowledge of anatomy and the mechanics of childbirth in terms of applied clinical knowledge, so you have to be explicit.

Teaching any skill can be broken down into a series of steps. The first is to demonstrate the skill to the trainee. Some methods suggest running through in silence so that the trainee can just observe the steps, and then repeating this while explaining what you are doing. In the Part 3 exam there is unlikely to be time to do this, so the best suggestion is to run through a demonstration while explaining what you are doing simultaneously. Ideally you should then ask the trainee to watch you doing the procedure while telling you what to do. Finally, they should be hands-on and do the procedure while explaining what they are doing. These three steps have been shown to be the best way to reinforce the steps of a procedure and promote understanding.

Time management is of the essence here. You only have ten minutes to potentially run through the scenario three times, and if props have been provided it is very important to allow the simulated junior doctor to have a chance to practise the skill. You should think of the common clinical skills that could be tested in this way and practise teaching these skills with your exam buddy so that you can go through the three steps in an unhurried way for common procedures. You will have seen that in the first video, the candidate passed the teaching skills even though she didn't follow the formal three steps, so the most important skill is time management to ensure you complete the task.

Giving feedback

Central to teaching a skill is giving feedback to the trainee in a formative way. There are a number of models for this. Each model includes a formula of identifying and reinforcing good behaviours or parts of the procedure that have been done well before moving on to discuss things that could have gone better. This is because starting a discussion with criticism is likely to result in a defensive attitude in the learner, meaning that the trainee is unlikely to take on board any constructive comments thereafter. Start by identifying good points and then proceed to discuss steps they could take to improve, or modifications to their technique to make a successful outcome more likely. Finally, summarise the good points again and make a plan for further development.

This doesn't have to be cumbersome or long-winded. It could be as simple as saying:

"You did really well in pulling in the correct direction, but I'd allow the head to descend a little more before changing the axis of traction to deliver the head. This was really good for a first attempt. Shall we try it again and this time I'll tell you when to change the direction of traction?"

While the candidate in video 2 did encourage the trainee to reflect on what they had done well and what could have been better, he didn't actually provide any feedback. The candidate in video 1 gave feedback as the task progressed, so you can see that you do not have to do everything strictly in the recommended order for teaching to pass the task. The examiners understand the time pressures on you in the exam and are looking for all the evidence that you know how to teach.

3. **Patient safety**

An instrumental delivery requires a good understanding of patient safety in a number of ways. First, informed consent is essential, so you should be able to explain and obtain verbal consent for a vacuum delivery. By convention, written consent is taken if proceeding to trial of vaginal delivery in theatre as those selected cases have been identified as being at higher risk of needing caesarean section. For a vacuum delivery in the delivery room, verbal consent is sufficient in the vast majority of cases.

Patients need to understand what is being done to them, so the competent candidate will explain to the ST1 trainee the need to keep talking to the patient, reassuring them, telling them what is being done and advising the patient when to 'push', 'pant' or rest.

The competent candidate will understand when an episiotomy is indicated to minimise the risk of a third-degree tear. They will explain to the ST1 trainee that it is important to check for a nuchal cord and to allow restitution of the head before delivering the body with the next contraction. They will then explain the need to deliver the placenta and repair any tears or the episiotomy and document the procedure clearly in the notes. Two other key elements of patient safety you should never forget are the estimation of blood loss and a swab and needle count at the beginning and end of the procedure.

Even if a vacuum delivery is anticipated to be straightforward and therefore is being done in the delivery room, there may be an unexpected failure of descent of the fetal head. The competent candidate will explain to the ST1 trainee when to abandon the procedure and proceed to caesarean section. You can do this during the procedure as you are allowing the simulated trainee to practise with the equipment; don't be tempted to spend too long just talking at the actor at the start of the task.

The final aspect of patient safety in the context of teaching a clinical skill is an overriding duty of care to the patient and the need to intervene if the patient is being put at risk. As you can see from this task, there are no tricks or hidden scenarios here, but it is entirely possible that the simulated trainee may have been instructed to do something incorrectly that would put a patient in danger. You need to be able to intervene and prevent harm without undermining or humiliating the trainee in this situation. There are no circumstances in which it is acceptable to shout at a junior colleague, so you need to practise being able to convey an urgent need to stop immediately without scaring the trainee (or the patient).

Don't be tempted to let the tutorial move on to a discussion about shoulder dystocia, retained placenta or repair of third-degree tears. Another key skill for the Part 3 exam is to be focused and specific. The instructions very clearly state teaching the technique of vacuum delivery, so going beyond this remit is more likely to result in a fail than a pass.

Summary

Teaching skills are regarded by both the RCOG and the GMC as being an essential core clinical skill for all doctors. In the Part 3 exam, a teaching task may appear to be a test of communication with colleagues, but is also a sophisticated test of interpersonal skills, an ability to provide leadership in a teaching situation, an awareness of patient safety and, above all, applied clinical knowledge. Knowing when or when not to do a procedure is as important as knowing how to do the procedure itself. Equally, being able to break down a procedure into its component parts in order to both explain it clearly and identify exactly which step a struggling trainee is having difficulty with is a key skill for you as a teacher.

While your patient is your first priority, your junior colleagues are also very important. We have a duty to pass on our clinical skills, but we must also do this in a kind and supportive way. It is important to correct technique or errors, but to do it in a way that acknowledges that, as their career progresses, they will become our peers rather than our subordinates, so they are owed respect while learning their craft. Remember, the word 'doctor' comes from the Latin word to teach, and passing on your skills is an integral part of the Hippocratic Oath.

Practise teaching skills with your exam buddy, including correcting mistakes and giving feedback using one of the methods given above. Try using a timer to practise doing this in ten minutes to mimic exam conditions.

Task 4: Retained Swab (Simulated Patient Task)

This task relates to module 8, postpartum problems (the puerperium) (core curriculum module 12).

Candidate's Instructions

This is a simulated patient task assessing:

- *information gathering*
- *communication with patients*
- *patient safety*
- *applied clinical knowledge.*

   You are on call for the Maternity Unit and are about to meet Ms Sofia Bryant-Smyth, who has presented late in the evening, having been delivered of her first baby two weeks previously.

   You have ten minutes in which you should:

- *establish the circumstances leading to the attendance*
- *manage the immediate situation*
- *advise on the immediate next steps to be taken*

If you have been working through each of the preceding three tasks, you will now be familiar with the instructions to spend two minutes thinking about how you would set about this task and make brief notes. Think about how you would approach this patient. It is late in the evening so there must be something fairly significant to bring a new mother back to the Maternity Unit rather than trying to settle her baby down for the night. Consider how you would establish a rapport with the patient and find out why she has come back to hospital so urgently that it could not wait until the next day. You should therefore assume she is likely to be distressed or upset and you should reflect on how to use a sympathetic approach to engage with her concerns as quickly as possible.

Now watch the two videos linked to the task. Make notes about the performance of the actor playing the role of the candidate in the core clinical skills that are being assessed in this task. For each of the clinical skills, decide whether the candidate's skills are at the level of a pass, fail or borderline.

After you have watched and scored this task, you can compare your assessment with the comments of trained Part 3 clinical and lay examiners. The aim of this process is to show you what behaviours are expected and to help you to understand how you will be assessed when you attempt the Part 3 examination.

Task 4, video 1: videos are hosted at www.cambridge.org/9781316627457

Video 1: Your Clinical Examiner Comments

Information Gathering

Comments:

Pass   Borderline   Fail

Communication with Patients

Comments:

Pass   Borderline   Fail

Patient Safety

Comments:

Pass   Borderline   Fail

Applied Clinical Knowledge

Comments:

Pass   Borderline   Fail

Now compare your comments and decisions with those of the clinical and lay examiners.

Video 1: Clinical Examiner's Comments

Information Gathering

Comments:

- Checks mode of delivery but mainly uses closed questions - 'are you generally well?' - not using specific questions, makes assumptions about not having temperatures.
- Does ask about abdominal pain, bleeding and discharge, but is not specific about symptoms and brushes over concerns.

Pass   (Borderline)   Fail

Communication with Patients

Comments:

- Does introduce herself but brusque attitude; seems dismissive of concerns - 'sometimes swabs get left behind'.
- Uses jargon - vagina, Datix form, risk management.
- Odd use of language 'cut and stitched up'.
- No empathy, apology appears superficial and insincere 'these things do happen'.
- Dismissive of concerns about breastfeeding on antibiotics.
- Doesn't address concerns about long-term effects.

Pass   (Borderline)   Fail

Patient Safety

Comments:

- Recognises need to send swab for histology and to take vaginal swabs and antibiotics.
- Confirms will report via Datix form and explains it is a 'never event'.
- Doesn't escalate to consultant on call or consultant she is booked under.

(Pass)   Borderline   Fail

Applied Clinical Knowledge

Comments:

- *Recognises need for swabs and antibiotics.*
- *Seems flustered by patient concerns, tries to dismiss concerns.*
- *Does apologise but doesn't make a management plan. No clear descrip-tion of risk management process and how patient will be contacted for debrief and formal apology.*
- *Becomes defensive when patient says she isn't happy; hasn't gained patient's trust that concerns will be dealt with.*
- *Self-taken swabs not appropriate in a patient with healing episiotomy, needs sensitive and careful examination; does recognise the importance of reassurance of a clinical examination.*

Pass   (Borderline)   Fail

Video 1: Lay Examiner Comments

Information Gathering

> **Comments:**
>
> - *Makes introduction but doesn't seem to be aware that the patient is upset and concerned.*
> - *Uses a lot of jargon, doesn't seem to take the patient's concerns seriously. Apologies don't seem genuine. Seems to avoid eye contact; very keen to take plastic bag from patient but isn't convincing that there won't be a cover up.*
> - *Seemed to close down discussion at a number of points.*
> - *Non-specific questions, seemed to make lots of assumptions based on very general enquiries.*

    Pass   Borderline    Fail

Communication with Patients

> **Comments:**
>
> - *Uses lots of jargon and doesn't explain process. Makes it difficult for patient to find out how to complain; is she trying to make sure the patient doesn't contact PALS?*
> - *Didn't address concerns about breastfeeding; didn't recognise that a new mum is most concerned about anything that could affect their baby.*
> - *Upbeat tone of voice makes it seem like a retained swab isn't a big deal and the patient shouldn't be concerned, despite saying it is a never event – disconnect between tone of voice and words spoken so appears untrustworthy.*

    Pass   Borderline   Fail

At first viewing, the video of the candidate seems to be a reasonable dialogue between a patient and doctor. However, really focusing on the non-verbal communication and what is actually said shows that this is a borderline fail task, with the lay examiner being very clear that they consider this to be a failing candidate. Remember the Part 3 exam has lay examiners for this very reason – they are trained to assess what you say from the perspective of a patient and her understanding of the clinical advice she is being offered. It is clear that clinical knowledge isn't the problem here; this candidate is a borderline fail due to their attitude and communication skills. This mirrors the GMC observation that most complaints relate to how doctors interact with their patient rather than clinical knowledge and skills.

Before you watch video 2, you may find it helpful to read the instructions given to the simulated patient. They are given detailed instructions so that their performance is consistent throughout the exam, ensuring that each candidate has the same opportunity to pass the task in all the areas assessed. The actor is given guidance about how the competent candidate should tackle the task. This may give you an insight into how the actor tries to help candidates by prompting them and asking questions. However, it is also very important to remember that the actor is allowed to react to what the candidate is saying so may become upset or angry if the candidate says or does something that is ill-advised or contrary to what the actor has been told would be good practice. No matter how angry the actor has been briefed to become, they won't shout or swear.

Simulated Patient's Instructions

You are Sofia Bryant-Smyth, a 35-year-old recruitment consultant living with James Murray, a research chemist. You gave birth to your daughter Lucinda two weeks ago in the Maternity Unit under the care of consultant obstetrician Mr Raja.

The pregnancy was uncomplicated but the labour at term was prolonged; a normal delivery followed with the help of an episiotomy. The episiotomy was repaired by the midwife and it seemed to take a long time for her to complete the exercise. At one point she asked a second midwife to check what she was doing.

You then went home the next day and were quite pleased that you had gone through the labour and delivery without any help from Mr Raja and his obstetric team, as the only contact you had was with the midwives.

You have been breastfeeding and there are no concerns about Lucinda.

This evening while taking a shower you felt something odd in the vaginal area and identified what seemed to be a piece of material. You tugged at it and eventually retrieved a very odd piece of material.

You showed your husband, who is very angry that this has happened and insisted that you return to the hospital immediately, taking the material with you. It is foul-smelling and you are not happy for the plastic bag to be opened. You are also not too keen to hand over what you think may be evidence of a mistake, but are willing to do so if the reasons are clearly explained to you. You are incensed that this could have happened, are worried that this will have caused you some harm and you not only want an explanation and an apology, but also to know what will happen to you now.

Please prevent the candidate from physically opening the plastic bag if they attempt to do so.

The clinical and lay examiners are instructed not to interact with the candidate or the simulated patient, but the clinical examiner can confirm that if the candidate offers to examine the patient, the pelvic findings on examination are unremarkable.

Now that you understand the actor's instructions, watch video 2 and score the second candidate in each of the four clinical skills domains.

Task 4, video 2: videos are hosted at www.cambridge.org/9781316627457

Video 2: Your Clinical Examiner Comments
Information Gathering

Comments:

Pass	Borderline	Fail

Communication with Patients

Comments:

Pass	Borderline	Fail

Patient Safety

Comments:

Pass	Borderline	Fail

Applied Clinical Knowledge

Comments:

Pass   Borderline   Fail

Compare your comments with those of the clinical and lay examiners.

Video 2: Clinical Examiner's Comments

Information Gathering

> **Comments:**
>
> - *Good signposting of consultation - 'Can I ask you some questions?' Detailed questioning, specific questions so patient is clear what information needed.*
> - *Checks details of delivery, postnatal course and breastfeeding. Gets details of clinical condition.*

    Pass   Borderline   Fail

Communication with Patients

> **Comments:**
>
> - *Adopts a very serious facial expression from the outset; seems to recognise seriousness of event.*
> - *Gives clear indication of how serious a retained swab is; engages with the patient and doesn't try to sweep issues under the carpet.*
> - *Open body language, excellent eye contact and apology forthcoming.*

Pass   Borderline   Fail

Patient Safety

> **Comments:**
>
> - *Seems to understand the risks of untreated infection and the need to screen with swabs and send item for further investigation.*
> - *Recognises that there is unlikely to be a long-lasting effect so provides authentic and believable reassurance to the patient.*

Pass   Borderline   Fail

Applied Clinical Knowledge

Comments:

- *Offers to examine, is clear about the nature of the examination and swabs needed.*
- *Proactive approach to examining the patient and taking swabs.*
- *Able to discuss the effect of antibiotics on breastfeeding; acknowledges patient safety issues of breastfeeding and antibiotic prescribing. Gives reassurance.*
- *Develops follow-up plan and summarises plan.*

(Pass)   Borderline   Fail

Video 2: Lay Examiner Comments

Information Gathering

> **Comments:**
> - *Really good body language, leaning forward, nodding, seems to be taking concerns seriously. Not scared to apologise and acknowledge a never event.*
> - *Lots of open questions, lets the patient guide the consultation.*

(**Pass**)   Borderline   Fail

Communication with Patients

> **Comments:**
> - *Signposts the consultation – 'Can I ask you some questions?'*
> - *Seems authentic, seems really concerned, not a defensive attitude.*
> - *Recognises patient's distress and concerns.*
> - *Happy to talk about concerns about breastfeeding.*

(**Pass**)   Borderline   Fail

It is worth reflecting on how different the actor's response is to both candidates. In the first case, it's clear that she didn't feel listened to or that her concerns were acknowledged, and on a couple of occasions she raised her voice (without shouting), showing that she hasn't felt that she has been listened to nor her concerns taken seriously. In the first video, she seems to question whether 'Dr Smith' will actually escalate this incident. Look at the two videos again and see how the simulated patient's response has been determined by the way the doctor has approached the consultation.

Learning Points

It is very important to recognise the need to apologise to this patient. A retained swab is termed a 'never event' as there can be no excuse for leaving a swab in a patient after a procedure. All instruments, swabs and sharps should be counted before and after every procedure, and if the count isn't correct, then the procedure isn't finished until a search is made and the missing item found, including X-raying the patient if necessary.

It is essential to apologise to the patient for the retained swab. This may seem unusual as the scenario makes it clear that the candidate wasn't involved in the patient's care at all, and it may seem logical that the midwife should be the one to apologise. This is the important principle of the 'duty of candour' that obligates clinicians to acknowledge that an untoward incident has occurred and to express regret and initiate a review of the incident by filling in an incident report to submit to the clinical governance team.

The apology is not an admission of guilt by the person offering the apology, it is a key part of being open and honest. There is good evidence that an early apology and recognition of something going wrong is likely to prevent rather than escalate litigation, so never be afraid to say sorry.

Read the Question

1. Establish the circumstances leading to the attendance

This is the information gathering part of the task and you will have to rely on using open questions as the scenario gives no suggestion as to the reason for the patient attending the maternity unit. Remember, in the exam you will not have the title of this section to guide you, so there will be no hint about the swab until you start talking to the actor. This should give you a clue that this task is not about a complex clinical case and you should use the two minutes standing outside the booth to focus on what communication skills you might need to use to deal with a distressed or angry patient out of hours. It's clearly important to be able to defuse the situation so that you can move on to the other parts of the task. Showing an empathic approach and being willing to apologise will rapidly calm the simulated patient down because the actor has been instructed to allow herself to be placated so that the candidate can move on through the scenario.

2. Manage the immediate situation

This part of the task focuses on patient safety. The competent candidate will have a good understanding of adverse event reporting structures and will recognise that in order to achieve a pass in the patient safety domain, they will have to describe those processes to the simulated patient. The use of the word 'immediate' means considering what you would do that evening. You will not be expected to describe the process of a detailed root cause analysis, but merely to explain that there will be a full investigation involving her, the results of which will then be shared with her and her partner. You would be expected to explain that you will submit an electronic clinical incident form, the 'Datix' form, to ensure that the clinical governance processes will automatically be triggered on the next working day.

3. Advise on the immediate next steps to be taken

This instruction gives the competent candidate the opportunity to demonstrate applied clinical knowledge by sending the swab to the histopathology department to ensure it is really a Raytec swab with a radio-opaque strip in it. The competent candidate will also recognise the need to examine the patient to check for further retained swabs and to take microbiology swabs. A course of appropriate antibiotics should be started and the competent candidate will demonstrate that they have a good understanding of prescribing in patients who are breastfeeding.

The competent candidate will start the discussion with the patient in an empathic manner, with a gentle approach using open questions. The simulated patient should be given time to talk and display her anger and the candidate should use their non-verbal communication skills to encourage this.

The candidate should then take back control of the situation by anticipating the patient's concerns – for example, about the effect of antibiotics and breast milk on her baby, and whether the incident might have caused long-term damage such as pelvic infection and subsequent reduction in fertility. This is a chance to show leadership skills by taking responsibility for reporting the incident and making a firm plan with the patient about how they will contact her to give her the results of the microbiology swabs and histology report.

Summary

The two videos relating to this task demonstrate how attitude can shape the actor's response to the same clinical situation. The first candidate appears to be trying to sweep the issues aside, whereas the second candidate recognises that this is a very serious incident, and while it is extremely unlikely that the patient will have suffered harm, it is nonetheless a serious incident and should be treated as such.

This should demonstrate to you that an understanding of clinical risk alone isn't sufficient to pass the Part 3 exam. You need to understand that how doctors talk to patients and their attitude and respect for patient's concerns will be an essential part of building a rapport with patients and agreeing a mutually acceptable plan of management.

6 Revision Resources

The practice of obstetrics and gynaecology is a huge subject which is constantly changing as applied clinical science informs our everyday practice. While this is an essential part of the application of evidence to routine practice, it can be daunting for the MRCOG candidate who just wants a firm curriculum from which to revise and which represents the sum total of knowledge to be tested in the examination. The reality is that the evidence base for clinical medicine is constantly evolving and, as reflective practitioners, we should all be keeping up to date with developing science.

The 'gestation period' for an exam question is 9–12 months, and while there is a clear need to cover all 14 modules tested in the Part 3 exam, it is natural for the exam committee to focus any questions on recent developments. Each question or task will be extensively reviewed and refined in exam committee meetings before being accepted as an appropriate question for the examination.

Hopefully the preceding chapters will have shown that trying to spot hot topics and only revising parts of the curriculum will put a candidate at high risk of failure. However, it is also true that new guidelines and developments will provide a fertile ground for writing new exam questions.

So, how should you approach exam revision?

Breadth Versus Depth

In order to pass the Part 2 written exam you need both breadth and depth for each module. The clinical skills are clearly defined in the curriculum. It is tempting to view the Part 3 exam as being purely about communication, but hopefully the practice resources contained in this book will have shown you that without sound clinical knowledge you won't be able to pass the exam. The starting point for revision is the core curriculum on the RCOG website.

In order to start working through each module in more depth, you should consider using the e-learning resources in StratOG.[1] There are resources covering core modules of the curriculum which are available free to trainees registered with the RCOG or for other doctors for a small fee. There are some topics which require in-depth understanding and for which detail is essential. This includes the guidelines relating to common

[1] https://stratog.rcog.org.uk

problems such as labour, delivery, hypertension in pregnancy, heavy menstrual bleeding and other common clinical problems that an ST5 could reasonably be expected to deal with on a daily basis. The standard to achieve a pass in these topics can be expected to be high, so you must have a good depth of knowledge for core clinical areas. Don't forget that the practice of obstetrics and gynaecology is probably subject to more laws in the UK than most other specialties, as in addition to laws like the *Mental Capacity Act* which affects all specialties, we also need to understand and adhere to the *Abortion Act*, *HFE Act* and Lord Fraser competency, as well as being aware of the illegal practice of female genital mutilation (FGM).

The Part 3 clinical skills assessment template (Appendix 1) is a useful guide to the types of task that might be used to assess the core clinical skills domains in each of the 14 modules.

Recent Publications

A new or updated publication by the RCOG will be an attractive resource for the exam committee to use to develop a new question or task, so it's worth reviewing which guidelines relevant to each of the modules have been recently posted on the RCOG website. The most obvious starting place is the Green-top Guidelines, which present both the summary guidance and also the evidence levels for each statement. However, don't just focus on Green-top Guidelines; there are also scientific impact statements, clinical governance advice, good practice documents, consent advice and patient information leaflets, all of which could be source material for a question or task. The Lindsay Stewart Centre for audit and clinical informatics delivers audits and clinical improvement projects on behalf of the RCOG, and there are a number of key peer-reviewed papers which can be accessed from their pages on the RCOG website.[2]

Reviews, Clinical Governance and Ethics Resources

Another useful resource is the RCOG CPD journal, *The Obstetrician and Gynaecologist*, or TOG as it is known. TOG articles for the preceding two years are free to Fellows and Members and to registered trainees. There are some articles that are free to view from the date of publication, or a subscription can be purchased. After two years the articles become open access and are free via the RCOG website. TOG articles are evidence-based reviews of practice and include ethical and clinical governance topics which can be hard to find in most research-based journals and publications. Given that these topics feature prominently in the Part 3 exam and may be novel concepts to junior trainees and those not working in the UK, these articles are a valuable revision resource.

[2] www.rcog.org.uk/en/guidelines-research-services/audit-quality-improvement/history-of-the-lindsay-stewart-centre-for-audit-and-clinical-informatics

Other Resources

The Cochrane Library is an online resource containing systematic reviews and meta-analyses of research for numerous clinical conditions and is a useful starting point for developing the skills of presenting the advantages and disadvantages of a management plan to a colleague or patient.[3] The reviews support healthcare decision-making and can be very useful in a structured discussion task.

The National Institute for Health and Care Excellence (NICE) is also an excellent resource and provides a very detailed discussion of the evidence that underpins the summary guidance which is often used to inform commissioning of clinical services by those managing the NHS budget. The guidelines are strongly evidence-based and provide detailed protocols about how to practise clinical medicine. These guidelines are daunting in their depth and detail, so a useful place to start is the NICE Pathways, which give clear stepwise advice about developing a clinical management plan. From the pathway you can identify gaps in your knowledge and then refer to the full guidance to deepen your knowledge. You will find that many of the NICE guidelines and Green-top Guidelines mirror each other, so you can be confident about the evidence base against which you are being assessed.

Research Papers

It's really important to recognise that there are essentially two types of paper published in the major peer-reviewed journals such as the *British Journal of Obstetrics and Gynaecology*, *Lancet* and *New England Journal of Medicine*. The first type includes reviews such as systematic reviews and meta-analyses, and statements from learned societies which should inform changes in practice. The second type is newly published research. The articles which publish the results of a research project are usually the start of an intellectual conversation either in correspondence or in subsequent projects which hope to confirm, build on or refute the results of the first publication. The importance of this is to realise that the former could be the basis for a question or task, but the first 'cutting-edge' paper about new research is unlikely to feature in the exam until the science underpinning the results is widely accepted and adopted. Therefore, during the six months of your revision for the MRCOG exam it is reasonable to be selective in your reading – after all, there are only 24 hours in each day.

Textbooks

Finally, don't we all love our textbooks? There are some aspects of clinical medicine that don't change because humans are evolving slowly (if at all). The textbooks of anatomy, physiology and to some extent pathology stay up to date for a very long time. While

---

[3] www.cochranelibrary.com/

these texts will underpin much of your revision for the Part 1 MRCOG exam, they will be less important for Parts 2 and 3, and this core knowledge will be assessed in a clinical setting as applied knowledge. Be honest with yourself and do a gap analysis of areas that you need to refresh, but try to be focused in re-reading these textbooks. Of course, this textbook is essential reading!

Conclusions

Hopefully this brief guide will serve as a starting point to direct you to important resources that can help you revise without overwhelming you. Be strategic in your reading and, above all, remember the advice in Chapter 4 about resilience, work–revision balance and looking after yourself.

Good luck in the Part 3 exam.

Appendix 1 Part 3 MRCOG Clinical Skills Assessment Template

The aim of the Part 3 examination is to assess the candidate's ability to demonstrate core clinical skills in the context of the skills, knowledge, attitudes and competencies as defined in the Part 2 MRCOG curriculum. This template defines the core clinical skills in relation to 14 knowledge-based modules that will be assessed in the Part 3 MRCOG examination.

The learning methods to acquire these skills are a combination of clinical teaching, summative and formative feedback via workplace-based assessments, reflective practice and formal teaching in local, regional and national courses.

The candidate will be expected to demonstrate the application of their clinical knowledge of obstetrics and gynaecology by their ability to:

- convey a sound and comprehensive evidence-based understanding of the Part 2 MRCOG curriculum in relation to the clinical tasks in the Part 3 examination
- justify investigations and interventions
- critically interpret clinical findings and results of investigations
- critically discuss management options and
- present a balanced view of the risks and benefits of interventions

Fundamental Communications Skills

The essential communication skills that underpin every patient–doctor interaction will be assessed in the context of all of the knowledge-based modules tested in the Part 3 examination. The candidate will be expected to demonstrate skills in:

- making an appropriate introduction giving their name, role, purpose of interaction, and establishing a rapport
- taking a concise, relevant history using a blend of mainly open and some closed questions, demonstrating a logical and clearly reasoned style of questioning
- empathy, active listening, responding to patient cues
- identifying and managing communication barriers including the use of interpreters
- giving information in manageable amounts using patient-friendly language, avoiding jargon and explaining clinical terms
- encouraging dialogue and shared decision-making

- negotiating skills but demonstrating respect for patient autonomy in decision-making, including when decisions are made against medical advice
- acknowledging and addressing patients' concerns
- taking informed consent, including an awareness of mental capacity
- maintaining patient dignity at all times
- ensuring appropriate use of chaperones for intimate examinations, maintaining dignity at all times and being sensitive to cultural and religious issues and
- adopting a non-judgemental approach to patients' concerns and decisions

Obstetricians and gynaecologists work within a clinical team and their abilities to communicate with all members of the team are fundamental elements of good medical practice and patient safety. The candidates will be expected to demonstrate skills in:

- communicating with colleagues verbally and legibly in written form, including an ordered approach to clinical information, documentation of positive and important negative findings and investigations ordered
- succinctly summarising clinical discussions and clinical decisions verbally and in written form
- an ordered approach to clinical and operation notes, discharge summaries, clinic letters and dealing with results and
- discussing difficult or sensitive issues with colleagues, such as clinical disagreement, errors, issues of probity or ill health

Module 1: Teaching

Learning outcome: to demonstrate core clinical skills in relation to teaching medical, midwifery and nursing colleagues and medical students.

Communicating with patients and families	Communicating with colleagues	Information gathering	Patient safety	Applied clinical knowledge
Appropriate introduction of self and learner to patient and family Ability to explain role of the learner and nature of interaction to patient and family Demonstrates an ability to obtain informed consent for teaching to take place from patient and family	Understands principles of adult learning and giving feedback Demonstrates appropriate steps in increasing clinical knowledge of the learner and in teaching a new skill Uses appropriate language and non-verbal language to encourage learning Invites questions and encourages dialogue Shows a logical approach to building on pre-existing skills of learner	Demonstrates an understanding of requirement to gauge needs and existing skills of learner Checks learning and understanding at appropriate intervals	Ensures that patient safety is maintained when teaching a practical skill, showing an understanding of when to continue teaching and when to intervene or halt the teaching session	Demonstrates an ability to teach evidence-based medicine, including an understanding of study design, evidence levels and appropriate interpretation of statistics Demonstrates knowledge of importance of learning objectives and outcomes in relation to topic being taught Demonstrates ability to conduct and give feedback on workplace-based assessments

Module 2: Core Surgical Skills

Learning outcome: to demonstrate core clinical skills in relation to surgical skills in both obstetrics and gynaecology.

Communicating with patients and families	Communicating with colleagues	Information gathering	Patient safety	Applied clinical knowledge
Demonstrates honesty where there is clinical uncertainty about surgical or management options	Ability to communicate legibly and with an ordered approach (date, time patient identification, etc.) e.g. clinical and operation notes	Demonstrates understanding of essential pre-operative investigations and relevant clinical assessment	Demonstrates understanding of principles of safe surgery including WHO safe surgery checklist	Knowledge in relation to obstetric and gynaecological surgery, including techniques and the risks and benefits of procedures
Ability to use non-directional counselling when advising patients of management options including no treatment	Demonstrates ability to teach appropriate skills to other colleagues in a logical and coherent manner with recognition of the learner, environment and resources available	Ability to interpret clinical findings and investigations when making decisions about surgical technique and approach	Demonstrates understanding of consent including consent of a child and the need to assess mental capacity in relation to consent	Demonstrates an ability to critically appraise medical media in relation to surgical procedures
	Ability to prioritise which cases are urgent and which can be dealt with later or electively	Ability to describe a clear action plan, including ongoing management plan after surgical procedure	Has an understanding of decision-making and consent for patients lacking capacity	Demonstrates an ability to weigh up pros and cons of surgical versus medical management of clinical conditions
			Demonstrates an understanding of moving and positioning the unconscious and recovering patient	Understanding of the appropriate use of blood products
			Recognises limits of their clinical abilities and demonstrates an understanding of when to call for help and involve senior colleagues and other disciplines	

Module 3: Post-Operative Care

Learning outcome: to demonstrate core clinical skills in relation to post-operative care for day-case patients, in-patients and those with significant co-morbidities or complications.

Communicating with patients and families	Communicating with colleagues	Information gathering	Patient safety	Applied clinical knowledge
Ability to provide psychological support for patients and their family Ability to discuss rehabilitation, discharge planning, recovery after discharge from hospital, return to work and follow-up Ability to describe a clear and logical action plan and rationale for follow-up	Ability to diagnose post-operative complications and formulate an appropriate management plan	Ability to request appropriate investigations and interpret those results Summarises discussions succinctly and checks patient understanding at appropriate intervals	Demonstrates an understanding of risk management and clinical governance processes in relation to post-operative complications Recognises limits of their clinical abilities and demonstrates an understanding of when to call for help and involve senior colleagues and other disciplines Demonstrates an understanding of safe prescribing in post-operative care, including recognition of drug interaction, allergies and special circumstances, e.g. renal impairment	Knowledge of the management of the post-operative patient, including fluid balance, analgesia, catheter management and wound healing Demonstrates understanding of the enhanced recovery programme and issues of post-operative rehabilitation Demonstrates understanding on the early and later risks of surgery and their amelioration

Module 4: Antenatal Care

Learning outcome: to demonstrate core clinical skills in relation to antenatal care.

Communicating with patients and families	Communicating with colleagues	Information gathering	Patient safety	Applied clinical knowledge
Ability to tackle difficult or sensitive topics including domestic violence, drug and alcohol abuse, child protection issues, female genital mutilation and honesty where there is clinical uncertainty Ability to discuss investigations, follow-up and plan for antenatal care Ability to succinctly summarise discussions with antenatal patients	A clear and logical approach to a differential diagnosis or management plan for antenatal patients Appropriate amount of detail to ensure management plans are clear and easily understood by colleagues Ability to communicate with colleagues in primary care, other specialities, e.g. obstetric anaesthetics and midwifery colleagues, including specialist midwives	Ability to take a concise and relevant antenatal history Skills in signposting and guiding the antenatal consultation Ensuring patient understanding and encouraging questions Ability to describe to the antenatal patient a clear action plan and the rationale for follow-up based on the discussion	Demonstrates ability to triage patient to different patterns of antenatal care according to risk factors Demonstrates awareness of safety of investigations and therapeutics during pregnancy, including safe prescribing Awareness of issues of drug and alcohol abuse, domestic violence and safeguarding Understanding of clinical governance and risk management for women declining usual antenatal care	Knowledge of antenatal care including PIH, IUGR, multiple pregnancy, prolonged pregnancy, VBAC and social and cultural factors Ability to interpret clinical examination findings and results of investigations in the context of the clinical scenario Awareness of the risks and benefits of various different management options balancing needs of the mother and fetus

Module 5: Maternal Medicine

Learning outcome: to demonstrate core clinical skills in relation to medical co-morbidities and complications of pregnancy.

Communicating with patients and families	Communicating with colleagues	Information gathering	Patient safety	Applied clinical knowledge
Ability to tackle difficult or sensitive topics including domestic violence, child protection issues and honesty where there is clinical uncertainty Gives information to the patient with co-existing medical disorders of both the impact of pregnancy on her pre-existing conditions and the impact of those conditions on the fetus	A clear and logical approach to a differential diagnosis or management plan for patients with medical disorders, both pre-existing and those arising in pregnancy Appropriate amount of detail to ensure management plans are clear and easily understood by colleagues Ability to communicate with colleagues in primary care and within the multidisciplinary team, including nurse specialists, physicians and psychiatrists	Ability to take a concise and relevant medical history Skills in signposting and guiding the consultation Ensuring patient understanding and encouraging questions Ability to describe to the patient with co-existing medical disorders a clear action plan and the rationale for follow-up based on the discussion	Demonstrates awareness of safety of investigations and therapeutics pre-conception, during pregnancy and in the postnatal period, including safe prescribing Demonstrates an understanding of both the impact of pregnancy on pre-existing conditions and the impact of those conditions on the fetus	Knowledge of pre-conception, antenatal and postnatal care, including the risks of maternal morbidity and mortality related to the medical co-morbidity

Module 6: Management of Labour

Learning outcome: to demonstrate core clinical skills in relation to management of normal and abnormal labour.

Communicating with patients and families	Communicating with colleagues	Information gathering	Patient safety	Applied clinical knowledge
Demonstrates an ability to communicate to the woman and her partner and/or family the interventions for abnormal labour and instrumental or operative delivery An ability to explain the risks and benefits of interventions for both the mother and the fetus	Makes clear the reason for the interaction with colleagues, e.g. handover Ability to prioritise cases appropriately into urgent, semi-urgent and non-urgent cases Ability to delegate tasks to colleagues and midwives appropriately Demonstrates understanding of limits of own competence and when to call for senior help or involve other specialties Demonstrates an ability to form a logical differential diagnosis for intrapartum complications and to be able to convey that to colleagues including when the consultant is off-site Appropriate amount of detail to ensure management plans are clear and easily understood by colleagues Demonstrates team working to support colleagues during peaks of activities on the labour ward Ability to teach appropriate skills to other colleagues in a logical and coherent manner with recognition of the learner, environment and resources available	Ability to synthesise a clear clinical picture from the patient, the notes, the partogram and information about the fetal heart in order to assess the clinical situation Ability to describe a clear action plan and rationale for decisions made based on the discussion	Awareness of patient safety in labour in different environments, e.g. water birth, birthing outside hospital Demonstrates understanding of risks from interventions such as regional analgesia, therapeutics in labour and invasive procedures Ensures use of chaperones for intimate examination Maintains patient dignity at all times Accurate prescribing in labour including management of intravenous infusions Acknowledges medical error, poor care or omissions and apologises as appropriate Demonstrates an understanding of risk management and clinical governance processes in relation to intrapartum care Ability to critically appraise intrapartum care in adverse events	Knowledge of intrapartum care including induction of labour, management of normal and abnormal labour, obstetric interventions, the interpretation of the CTG Ability to critically appraise medical media including guidelines, protocols and scientific papers Demonstrates an ability to think and work under pressure from competing priorities when the workload on the labour ward is heavy Demonstrates a working knowledge of the roles and responsibilities of other members of the multidisciplinary team Demonstrates an ability to appropriately delegate tasks when the workload on the labour ward requires

Module 7: Management of Delivery

Learning outcome: to demonstrate core clinical skills in management of normal delivery, operative delivery and third stage.

Communicating with patients and families	Communicating with colleagues	Information gathering	Patient safety	Applied clinical knowledge
Gains verbal or written consent for intervention or operative delivery	Ability to prioritise cases requiring delivery, including understanding of categories of caesarean section	Demonstrates ability to interpret notes on progress of labour, partogram and findings on vaginal examination in order to decide on management of delivery, both second and third stages	Demonstrates understanding of principles of safe surgery for operative delivery, including WHO safe surgery checklist	Knowledge of management of delivery including preterm delivery, management of malposition and malpresentation and multiple pregnancy
	Demonstrates an ability to formulate an appropriate management plan for delivery	Ability to describe a clear action plan for management of delivery	Demonstrates appropriate prioritisation throughout	Ability to demonstrate clinical, technical and operative skills
	Demonstrates an understanding of the roles of the multidisciplinary team, including liaison with laboratory colleagues in dealing with massive obstetric haemorrhage, liaison with neonatal team and other centres		Acknowledges medical error, omission or poor care and apologises as appropriate	Demonstrates a working knowledge of the roles and responsibilities of other members of the multidisciplinary team
	Ability to communicate verbally with the multidisciplinary team, including anaesthetists, theatre staff and neonatologists, in an efficient and timely manner		Demonstrates an understanding of risk management and clinical governance processes in relation to management of delivery	Demonstrates understanding of neonatal networks and need to transfer to tertiary units
	Demonstrates ability to teach appropriate skills to other colleagues in a logical and coherent manner with recognition of the learner, environment and resources available		Ability to critically appraise management of delivery in adverse events	

Module 8: Postpartum Problems (The Puerperium)

Learning outcome: to demonstrate core clinical skills in relation to postnatal care.

Communicating with patients and families	Communicating with colleagues	Information gathering	Patient safety	Applied clinical knowledge
Ability to tackle difficult or sensitive topics including domestic violence, child protection issues and honesty where there is clinical uncertainty Ability to describe to the postnatal patient a clear action plan and the rationale for follow-up based on the discussion	A clear and logical approach to a differential diagnosis or management plan for postnatal patients Appropriate amount of detail to ensure management plans are clear and easily understood by colleagues Ability to communicate with colleagues in primary care and other specialities, e.g. obstetric anaesthetics, neonatologists, physicians, microbiologists and midwifery colleagues, including specialist midwives, perinatal mental health specialists and community midwives	Ability to take a concise and relevant postnatal history Skills in signposting and guiding the postnatal consultation Ensuring patient understanding and encouraging questions Ability to succinctly summarise discussions with the postnatal patient	Demonstrates awareness of safety of investigations and therapeutics during the postnatal period and during lactation, including safe prescribing Understanding of safeguarding issues for neonate and vulnerable adults Understanding of psychological co-morbidities including puerperal psychosis and risk of self-harm	Knowledge of postnatal care including the risks of maternal morbidity, mortality and psychiatric disorders related to the postnatal period Ability to recognise the critically ill or deteriorating patient and apply an evidence-based approach to management of postpartum complications

Module 9: Gynaecological Problems

Learning outcome: to demonstrate the core clinical skills in relation to gynaecological conditions.

Communicating with patients and families	Communicating with colleagues	Information gathering	Patient safety	Applied clinical knowledge
Gives information in manageable amounts regarding information, investigations, diagnoses and management of gynaecological problems Ability to describe a clear and logical action plan and rationale for follow-up	Ability to prioritise cases appropriately Ability to describe the differential diagnosis and formulate an appropriate management plan	Demonstrates ability to take a comprehensive history from patients and their families Demonstrates a logical and clearly reasoned style of questioning Ability to request appropriate investigations and interpret those results and operative findings in order to develop a clear management plan and rationale for follow-up Summarises discussions succinctly and checks patient understanding at appropriate intervals	Demonstrates an understanding of risk management and clinical governance processes in relation to gynaecological disorders Recognises limits of their clinical abilities and demonstrates an understanding of when to call for help and involve senior colleagues and other disciplines Demonstrates an understanding of safe prescribing in gynaecological disorders, including recognition of drug interaction, allergies and special circumstances, e.g. renal impairment Demonstrates understanding of principles of safe surgery, including WHO safe surgery checklist	Knowledge of the treatment of gynaecological disorders including menstrual disorders, endocrine disorders, disorders of puberty, congenital anomalies, the climacteric and emergency gynaecology Demonstrates an ability to critically appraise medical media in relation to gynaecological treatment Demonstrates understanding of the role of imaging in gynaecological disorders Understanding of referral pathways for gynaecological disorders Demonstrates ability to take informed consent, including assessment of mental capacity Demonstrates ability to present management options and their risks and benefits using non-directional counselling

Module 10: Subfertility

Learning outcome: to demonstrate core clinical skills in relation to couples with a history of subfertility.

Communicating with patients and families	Communicating with colleagues	Information gathering	Patient safety	Applied clinical knowledge
Gives information about infertility, investigations and treatments in manageable amounts using patient-friendly language, avoiding jargon	Ability to describe the differential diagnosis and formulate an appropriate management plan	Demonstrates ability to take a comprehensive history from both partners of an infertile couple	Demonstrates an understanding of risk management and clinical governance and regulatory processes in relation to infertility, including issues of confidentiality	Knowledge of the treatment of infertility, including surgical management of tubal disease, endometriosis and male infertility
Demonstrates honesty around benefits, side-effects, complications and outcomes of fertility treatments		Ability to request appropriate investigations and interpret those results from both female and male partners and operative findings in order to develop a clear management plan and rationale for follow-up	Understanding of the need to consider the welfare of the child in providing fertility treatments	Demonstrates sound evidence-based clinical knowledge of ovulation induction, assisted conception and gamete donation, including the risks and limitations of these treatments
Demonstrates an understanding of the psychological needs of the partner as well as the infertile woman		Summarises discussions succinctly and checks patient understanding at appropriate intervals	Understanding of the risks of multiple pregnancy associated with fertility treatments	Demonstrates an ability to critically appraise medical media in relation to infertility treatments
Understanding of the psychological issues and sensitivities surrounding infertility				Demonstrates an understanding of the role of the HFEA and the NHS funding restrictions and rationing of assisted conception
				Understanding of the role of counselling for the infertile couple
				Understanding of cultural issues and issues relating to same-sex partners and single parents

Module 11: Sexual and Reproductive Health

Learning outcome: to demonstrate core clinical skills in relation to contraception, termination of pregnancy and sexual health, including legal and ethical issues.

Communicating with patients and families	Communicating with colleagues	Information gathering	Patient safety	Applied clinical knowledge
Demonstrates tact, empathy, concern and respect for patients and maintains patient dignity at all times Demonstrates a non-judgemental attitude when caring for patients Demonstrates the ability to communicate with teenagers and encourages them to involve parents/guardians Demonstrates respect for beliefs, values and sexual diversity Ability to describe a clear and logical action plan and rationale for follow-up	Ability to prioritise cases appropriately Ability to describe the differential diagnosis and formulate an appropriate management plan	Demonstrates ability to take a comprehensive sexual health history Ability to request appropriate investigations and interpret those results and operative findings in order to develop a clear management plan and rationale for follow-up Summarises discussions succinctly and checks patient understanding at appropriate intervals	Demonstrates an understanding of risk management and clinical governance processes in relation to sexual and reproductive health Demonstrates an understanding of safe prescribing, including recognition of drug interaction, allergies and special circumstances, e.g. renal impairment	Knowledge of sexual and reproductive health including contraception, UK MEC guidelines, unplanned pregnancy and sexually transmitted infections Demonstrates understanding of the laws in relation to termination of pregnancy, STIs, consent, child protection and the *Sexual Offences Act 2003* Understanding of the roles and responsibilities of counsellors, police, primary care, social workers, GUM specialists and the voluntary sector in sexual and reproductive health

Module 12: Early Pregnancy Care

Learning outcome: to demonstrate core clinical skills in relation to the diagnosis, management and follow-up of complications of early pregnancy

Communicating with patients and families	Communicating with colleagues	Information gathering	Patient safety	Applied clinical knowledge
Empathic approach to bereavement of early pregnancy loss and the effect on both partners Ability to describe a clear and logical action plan and rationale for follow-up	Ability to prioritise cases appropriately Ability to describe the differential diagnosis and formulate an appropriate management plan	Demonstrates ability to take a comprehensive history Ability to request appropriate investigations and interpret those results and operative findings in order to develop a clear management plan and rationale for follow-up Summarises discussions succinctly and checks patient understanding at appropriate intervals	Demonstrates an understanding of risk management and clinical governance processes in relation to disorders of early pregnancy Recognises limits of their clinical abilities and demonstrates an understanding of when to call for help and involve senior colleagues and other disciplines Demonstrates an understanding of safe prescribing in early pregnancy, including recognition of drug interaction, allergies and special circumstances, e.g. renal impairment Demonstrates understanding of principles of safe surgery, including WHO safe surgery checklist	Knowledge of early pregnancy complications including trophoblastic disease, ectopic pregnancy and recurrent miscarriage Understanding of surgical techniques for managing early pregnancy complications Demonstrates an ability to critically appraise medical media in relation to early pregnancy disorders Demonstrates ability to present management options and their risks and benefits using non-directional counselling Demonstrates understanding of the impacts of early pregnancy problems on future fertility and outcomes in future pregnancy

Module 13: Gynaecological Oncology

Learning outcome: to demonstrate core clinical skills in relation to the screening, diagnosis, management and palliation of gynaecological malignancies.

Communicating with patients and families	Communicating with colleagues	Information gathering	Patient safety	Applied clinical knowledge
Gives information in manageable amounts to the patient and her family regarding investigations, diagnoses and management of gynaecological malignancies Demonstrates ability to deal sensitively with palliation and death Ability to describe a clear and logical action plan	Ability to prioritise cases appropriately Ability to describe the differential diagnosis and formulate an appropriate management plan	Demonstrates ability to take a comprehensive gynaecological oncology history from patients and their families Ability to request appropriate investigations and interpret those results and operative findings in order to develop a clear management plan and rationale for follow-up Summarises discussions succinctly and checks patient understanding at appropriate intervals	Understanding of the referral pathways and targets for investigation and treatment of gynaecological cancers Demonstrates an understanding of risk management and clinical governance processes in relation to gynaecological cancers Recognises limits of their clinical abilities and demonstrates an understanding of when to call for help and involve senior colleagues and other disciplines Demonstrates an understanding of safe prescribing in gynaecological disorders, including recognition of drug interaction, allergies and special circumstances, e.g. renal impairment Demonstrates understanding of principles of safe surgery, including WHO safe surgery checklist	Knowledge of the epidemiology, presentation, investigation and treatment of gynaecological malignancies, including palliation Understanding of roles and responsibilities of the members of the multidisciplinary team Demonstrates an ability to critically appraise medical media in relation to gynaecological cancers Demonstrates understanding of the role of screening and imaging in gynaecological malignancies Understanding of referral pathways for gynaecological cancers Demonstrates ability to present management options and their risks and benefits using non-directional counselling

Module 14: Urogynaecology and Pelvic Floor Problems

Learning outcome: to demonstrate core clinical skills in relation to urogynaecological disorders including incontinence and pelvic organ prolapse.

Communicating with patients and families	Communicating with colleagues	Information gathering	Patient safety	Applied clinical knowledge
Gives information about urogynaecological examination, investigations and treatments in manageable amounts using patient-friendly language, avoiding jargon Demonstrates honesty around benefits, side-effects, complications and clinical uncertainty about long-term outcomes of urogynaecological treatments Understanding of the psychological issues and sensitivities surrounding urogynaecological disorders and incontinence	Ability to describe the differential diagnosis and formulate an appropriate management plan Ability to clearly communicate requirements and situation with theatre staff, assistants and anaesthetists	Ability to take a comprehensive urogynaecological history Ability to interpret urodynamic investigations, microbiological reports, cystometry, imaging and fluid balance charts in order to reach a diagnosis and develop a management plan	Demonstrates understanding of principles of safe surgery, including WHO safe surgery checklist Demonstrates an understanding of safe prescribing in relation to urogynaecological therapeutics Demonstrates an understanding of the contraindications and interactions of urogynaecological drugs and common medical treatments and co-morbidities	Knowledge of the surgical, non-surgical and medical management of urogynaecological disorders, including pelvic organ prolapse, acute voiding disorders, over-active bladder and stress urinary incontinence Demonstrates an ability to critically appraise medical media in relation to urogynaecological treatments Demonstrates an ability to weigh up pros and cons of surgical versus medical management of urogynaecological disorders

Index